Distinguishing Psychological from Organic Disorders

Robert L. Taylor, M.D., is Medical Director of the Austin-Travis County MHMR Center in Austin, Texas.

Distinguishing Psychological from Organic Disorders

Screening for Psychological Masquerade

Robert L. Taylor, M.D.

Springer Publishing Company

Copyright © 1990 by Robert L. Taylor, M.D.

All rights reserved

Published by Springer Publishing Company.

This is a new edition of a book published by McGraw-Hill in 1982 entitled
MIND OR BODY: DISTINGUISHING PSYCHOLOGICAL FROM ORGANIC DISORDERS,
© 1982 Robert L. Taylor, M.D.

No part of this publication may be reproduced, stored in a
retrieval system, or transmitted in any form or by any means,
electronic, mechanical, photocopying, recording, or otherwise,
without the prior permission of Springer Publishing Company, Inc.

Springer Publishing Company, Inc.
536 Broadway
New York, NY 10012

91 92 93 94 / 5 4 3

Library of Congress Cataloging-in-Publication Data

Taylor, Robert L., 1942–
    Distinguishing psychological from organic disorders : screening
for psychological masquerade / Robert L. Taylor.
        p.   cm.
    Includes bibliographical references.
    ISBN 0-8261-6950-3
    1. Mental illness—Physiological aspects.   2. Psychological
manifestations of general diseases.   3. Diagnosis, Differential.
4. Neuropsychiatry.   I. Title.
    [DNLM: 1. Mental Disorders—diagnosis.   2. Organic Mental
Disorders—diagnosis.   WM 141 T244d]
RC455.4.B5T38   1990
616.89′075—dc20
DNLM/DLC
for Library of Congress   90-9477
                                                                                CIP

For information about our audio products, write us at:
Newbridge Book Clubs, 3000 Cindel Drive, Delran, NJ   08370

To
Lester and Mary Lou Taylor

and to
Vanessa and Abbott

CONTENTS

PREFACE

The personal encounters we have in our everyday lives can create striking changes in the way we think, feel, and act. But such changes are not invariably related to external events; sometimes, they are the unrecognized product of an underlying physical disease. In these instances, despite having a psychological appearance, the symptoms reflect a breakdown in the brain itself; a breakdown that is not amenable to psychological therapies.

Distinguishing masquerading medical conditions from psychological problems is an ongoing challenge for all therapists and counselors. The stakes are considerable. Errors in this critical clinical assessment lead to frustration, inappropriate therapy, and, in more tragic cases, residual disability and even death. Few moments are more distressing than when a therapist finds that a patient whose symptoms have been construed as expressions of psychological conflict is, in fact, suffering from a brain tumor, seizure disorder, or some other organic condition.

This book is a practical guide to the clinical recognition of *psychological masquerades that result from a variety of organic mental disorders.* Illustrative case histories, drawn primarily from published accounts, are interwoven with general principles. Instead of an encyclopedic detailing of every medical disease known to cause psychiatric symptoms, the book provides the reader with a basic approach that, if applied consistently, reduces the chances of mistaking organic disorders for psychological problems.

I want to express special thanks to Larry Koran who several years ago set me to seriously thinking about the subject of this book and who thoughtfully reviewed the early draft chapters.

I am grateful to Barbara Arons and the staff of the inpatient psychiatric service at Santa Clara Valley Medical Center (San Jose, California) from whom I learned invaluable lessons with respect to the clinical recognition of psychological masquerade.

For their published accounts of masquerading organic disorders I am also indebted to various authors—most of whom I have never met.

Finally, the book has been improved considerably in response to comments from Frank Benson, Pat Jordan, Bev Abbot, David Lam, Linda Olvera-Perales, Lenore Morell, and Merna McMillan.

Chapter 1

Appearances Can Be Deceiving

Difficulties lie in our habits of thought rather than in the nature of things.   —Andre Tardieu

Psychiatric symptoms are not always best explained psychologically. Mental and emotional changes commonly associated with various problems in living can result from dysfunctions within the body itself. This creates a problem in clinical assessment. Is the patient depressed because of a job failure or loss of a lover; or is the depression a manifestation of hormonal imbalance, brain tumor, or epilepsy?

Certain organic disorders have an uncanny potential for producing symptoms easily misconstrued as nonmedical conditions; in short, they masquerade. They tend to mislead the professionals who struggle to understand their true nature. The challenge of recognizing these psychological masquerades cannot be dismissed by the nonmedically trained professional as a "medical task." Patients do not automatically find their way to the most appropriate service facility.

Psychological masquerade is the "flip-side" of the psychosomatic complaint. Just as individuals with problems in living sometimes inappropriately seek the care of physicians, persons with brain disease sometimes look for cures from psychotherapists. Like it or not, all mental health professionals are confronted with the task of clinically distinguishing psychological reactions from organic mental disorders. As we shall see, these misleading presentations are not uncommon; and, often, they appear in the context of a plausible life stress or conflict, further complicating their clinical recognition.

The task of detecting psychological masquerade cannot be avoided. It can be bungled, but not avoided. Clear distinctions between medical and nonmedical responsibility occur only on organizational charts and in the

1

pages of job descriptions and textbooks. In the everyday world, the boundaries are blurred. Mastering the clinical skills and knowledge necessary to minimize the chances of misinterpreting organic mental disorders is the responsibility of all mental health professionals. They owe this to themselves as professionals and more importantly, to their patients.

For the nonmedically trained professional, assessing for psychological masquerade does not require an indepth knowledge of neurology. Arriving at a specific diagnosis is the role of medical specialists. What is needed is the clinical ability to *suspect* organicity so that referral for further medical evaluation can be made.

STORY OF TWO LANGUAGES

Throughout this book we will contrast psychological reactions with organic mental disorders. At times the discussion may seem overly simplistic, characterizing mental and emotional reactions as either organic or psychological in nature. Actually, human problems are neither organic nor psychological! It is the language we choose to explain a given problem that is "organic" or "psychological." If our knowledge of human behavior were complete, one all-encompassing language would suffice. As it is, various "partial" languages or models are used to explain problems. Among the disciplines primarily concerned with explaining human behavior, two languages are commonly used. For convenience we will call them Language I and Language II.

Language I is mechanistic in character. It is used in the physical and biological sciences because of its capacity for communicating with considerable specificity. In contrast, Language II is much more subjective and metaphorical. It is widely used in the arts and social sciences due to its potential for expressing motivation, meaning, and feeling.

Psychological reactions to problems in living are much more readily described in Language II than in Language I. Consequently, explanations for these reactions are characteristically framed as psychological hypotheses. The man is depressed because he did not get the position at work. The loss is a blow to his self-esteem which leads to a sense of despondency. This explanation suggests such nonbiological remedies as acquiring another job or exploring his self-image in psychotherapy.

Language II is not nearly as useful with respect to other kinds of problems, however. For example, it is relatively unproductive in describing and providing a useful understanding of abdominal pain associated with appendicitis or peptic ulcer. In contrast, physiological explanations stated in Language I lead to effective treatments like surgical intervention or the use of histamine-blocking medication. This not to say that Language II could not be used to describe abdominal pain; it is just that the forthcoming solutions would not be as effective as those stemming from Language I. The opposite would be true with respect to other types of problems.

An explanation of human grief stated in biochemical terms using Language I would be cumbersome and rather limited in practical insights and productive solutions; not so with Language II. The point is this: any human problem can be explained in either organic (Language I) or psychological (Language II) terms. *The choice of one language over the other should depend on which will provide the more useful basis for productive solutions.* This book is concerned with those symptoms that are typically described in psychological terms but sometimes require a biological conceptualization. Errors in this aspect of clinical judgment set the stage for treating brain tumor as a personality disturbance, thyroid disease as an anxiety disorder, or brain seizure as psychosis.

Failure to identify organic mental disorders causes unnecessary expense, inappropriate treatment, patient frustration, and, in some cases, even death.

> A college senior experienced a sensation of pressure in her head. Following graduation, she found herself becoming easily upset about minor problems arising in her new job as a school teacher. In a short time she had lost fifteen pounds and had no appetite. She sought the help of a psychiatrist, who diagnosed her condition as schizophrenia.
>
> Subsequently, after suffering fainting episodes, vomiting, and unexplained fever, she underwent a complete medical evaluation. No physical basis for her symptoms could be found.
>
> Although her symptoms gradually disappeared without treatment, the woman began to act peculiarly. Despite electroconvulsive treatment, she became increasingly delusional and, finally, was admitted to a psychiatric hospital. She was described as "silly," alternating between periods of euphoric excitement and withdrawn depression. On occasion she expressed concern over what she feared was her impending death.
>
> Her admitting psychiatric diagnosis was hebephrenic schizophrenia. (Rupert & Remington, 1962)

Later, the diagnosis was questioned. On the basis of rapidly emerging neurological findings, surgery was performed and revealed a large frontal lobe brain tumor. Even though the tumor was not malignant, due to its advanced stage, it could not be successfully removed. The patient died.

This failure to recognize psychological masquerade resulted in death that could have been avoided had the organic condition been suspected earlier.

PSYCHOLOGICAL MASQUERADERS: HOW COMMON ARE THEY?

Over the years various researchers have tried to determine the frequency of psychological masquerade. One well-designed research investigation took a careful look at 658 consecutive psychiatric outpatient cases for evidence of "medical disorders productive of psychiatric symptoms." All the individuals had sought help for what they believed to be psychological problems. But in 9% of the cases the person had an organic disorder that fully accounted for the presenting "psychological" problem. The researchers concluded: "Psychiatric symptoms are nonspecific and commonly occur in medical as well as psychiatric disease" (Hall, Popkin, DeVaul, Faillace & Stickney, 1978).

Another somewhat larger study of 2,090 psychiatric outpatients turned up an even higher incidence of medical problems masquerading as psychiatric symptoms: 18% of the patients had symptoms directly attributable to organic disease. The author of the report emphasized the importance of persistent vigilance by clinicians: "The examiner must continually entertain the questions: What other than the obvious might be the cause of or a contributing factor to the presenting symptom" (Koranyi, 1979).

More recently (1983–1984), under a contract with the California Department of Mental Health, Dr. Lorrin Koran of Stanford University's Department of Psychiatry and his colleagues used a specially designed mobile evaluation unit to examine 529 patients drawn from eight program categories in the state's public mental health system (Koran et al., 1989). Underlying organic conditions either causing or significantly exacerbating the mental or emotional symptoms were found in 17% of the cases. Roughly half of the subjects who were approached, however, were not included in the study. They refused or were either too violent or psychotic to cooperate; or, they had a primary diagnosis of alcoholism. Because psychological masquerade is overrepresented in these types of subjects, the figure of 17% likely is on the low side.

In the report of these findings to the California Department of Mental Health, nine additional studies were summarized. Taking these ten studies together, the average occurrence of psychological masquerade was 19%.

Using a reverse approach, a group of researchers focused on 395 neurology patients, all of whom had well-documented organic disease. They posed this question: Initially, how many of these cases were erroneously thought to be psychological reactions? To find an answer, the researchers conducted an extensive review of the medical records. It showed that 53 (13%) of these patients had been diagnosed originally as having a psychological problem. The mistaken diagnoses included hysteria, schizophrenia, hypochondriasis, psychopathic personality, obsessive compulsive neurosis, anxiety, and somatization. On the average these false diagnoses had been maintained for four years. At one time or another over the course of their illnesses, all of these patients had received psychotherapy for symptoms that eventually were accounted for on a neurological basis (Tissenbaum, Harter, & Friedman, 1951).

Certain symptoms that traditionally have been characterized as "psychological," in light of new evidence, require much closer scrutiny. For example, it was not too long ago that mental health professionals were taught that male sexual impotence was almost always a psychological problem. This turns out not to be the case; most often, the cause is organic.

In a report appearing in the *Journal of the American Medical Association*, roughly 75% of 105 men studied were found to have physical diseases such as diabetes mellitus or specific sex-hormone imbalance, or to use drugs which were likely causes of their impotence (Spark, White & Connolly, 1980). Of the 34 men with hormonal problems who accepted treatment, 33 had a return of sexual potency. In an attempt to correct the problem, fourteen of these men had undergone psychotherapy unsuccessfully.

"Hysteria" is another psychological characterization not to be applied prematurely. One investigation followed 85 persons who under the examining eyes of experienced physicians were presumed to have hysteria, characterized by somatic complaints without demonstrable organic disease and thought to be the manifestation of psychological conflict (Slater, 1965). These patients were followed for periods ranging from 7 to 11 years. During this time more than one-third proved to have organic diseases that accounted for their "hysterical" symptoms.

Psychological masquerade commonly occurs in psychiatric inpatient populations. A review of "100 patients of lower socioeconomic class" admitted to a state hospital showed that 46% of the patients had medical illnesses that "directly caused or greatly exacerbated their symptoms." This determination was made on the basis of an extensive diagnostic evaluation, including physical, psychiatric, and neurological examinations along with an automated blood analysis and complete blood count, urinalysis, electrocardiogram, and sleep-deprived electroencephalogram. An additional 34% were found to have previously unrecognized physical illnesses, that (although not causative of psychiatric symptoms) "would have routinely been treated by a general physician if its presence were known" (Hall, Gardner, Stickney, LeCann, & Popkin, 1980).

These selected studies make it clear that psychological masquerade is by no means rare. Conservatively, one can assume that among psychiatric outpatients at least 10% of persons seen for psychological symptoms, if adequately evaluated will be found to suffer from a causative or contributing organic disease. These problems are often completely resolved by treating the organic disease. The figure of 10% for organic masqueraders increases as we move from outpatient to inpatient and emergency settings. Similarly, the 10% figure is increased in certain high risk populations, such as the elderly, and among diagnostic categories such as hysteria, sexual impotence, and drug/alcohol problems.

These findings do not change the basic fact that the majority of cases exhibiting mental or emotional symptoms are appropriately explained psychosocially. They do indicate, however, that any mental health professional actively engaged in clinical work can expect to see a significant number of masquerading medical conditions over the course of a career.

HOW *NOT* TO DETECT PSYCHOLOGICAL MASQUERADE

A sound approach to clinical assessment is based on the understanding that organic mental disorders and psychological reactions *are not primarily distinguishable* by the characteristics of the mental and emotional symptoms themselves.

It is the broader clinical context—the client's history as well as other clinical observations—that provides the most reliable basis for detecting psychological masquerade.

Consider the following case:

> Somewhat unwillingly, a 42-year-old man—the proprietor of a small grocery store in a rural area—was brought for treatment by his wife and brother. They stated that he had become highly irresponsible, engaging in impulsive and extravagant business deals.
>
> Further history revealed that the man had been a respected member of his community for many years. Although described as having his faults (such as boasting and ostentatious spending of money from time to time), he had been a responsible husband-provider with no history of mental illness. Over the past year, however, his wife had noticed several striking changes. He had become extremely forgetful and prone to spells of unexplained anger. At other times his mood would shift abruptly to one of euphoria. During these periods the man would indulge in wild spending sprees and become preoccupied with fantastic schemes. In recent months he had neglected his grocery-store business, spending much of his time driving about the countryside looking for new places to build bigger stores.

Finally, when he impulsively purchased an automobile and the following day solicited a large loan from the town banker at the conclusion of church services, his wife was convinced of his need for professional help. As he tried to persuade the banker of the merits of his proposal, he had gotten quite excited, to the point of becoming incoherent.

A clinical evaluation confirmed the man's inappropriate euphoria. He also showed a notable inability to perform simple math problems and to grasp commonly used proverbs. (Hofling, 1968)

The changes could have been psychological. Here was a man in his mid-forties, possibly confronting the meaning of his life, unable to avoid the inevitability of aging and eventual death. Construing this man's problem as a mid-life crisis would not have been unreasonable. Irrational, impulsive behavior does occur in response to stress. On closer examination, however, a psychological explanation was questionable. There were two major clues to an organic cause: serious difficulty performing simple calculations, particularly unexpected in a man who owned his own grocery store and the absence of any previous history of manic behavior. (Additionally, when examined medically, the man's pupils were found to be abnormally constricted and barely reactive to light.) Later, a blood test for syphilis was strongly positive, leading to a diagnosis of syphilitic brain disease. Additional history confirmed an untreated chancre sore during adolescence.

He was treated with high doses of intramuscular penicillin and after 6 weeks showed virtually complete recovery, a fortunate and somewhat unusual therapeutic response for someone with advanced (tertiary) syphilis.

The hypomanic behavior this man evidenced was no different than that experienced by persons with bipolar disorder or as a side effect to certain medications. The key to suspecting a psychological masquerade was not his euphoric, impulsive behavior. It was the cognitive deficit—his inability to solve simple math problems—that provided the most telling clinical finding.

WE SEE WHAT WE LOOK FOR

Distinguishing between organic and psychological disorders is complicated by our fixed patterns of perception—our mind set. Words and concepts help to organize the world around us; they also powerfully circumscribe what we perceive. For example, people who live most of their lives surrounded by snow learn to distinguish many different kinds, whereas a visitor may have difficulty discerning more than a single variety. This phenomenon is also at work as we evaluate problems clinically. All clinicians develop favorite explanations for various kinds of behavior. We become attached to them, sometimes to the extent that they adversely affect the clinical observations we make. Evidence supporting our preconceived ideas may be selectively recorded while contradictory findings are ignored, both forms of distortion occurring outside our conscious awareness. If this tendency becomes exaggerated, it is not long before we are viewing almost every case as another instance of "repressed anger" or "primary narcissism" or "neurotransmitter imbalance." Although clinical hypotheses provide a valuable function by allowing us to organize our clinical observations, they also create blind spots (Abercrombie, 1960).

In G.K. Chesterton's *The Invisible Man*, one of the characters, sensing that murder is intended, sends four men to keep watch over the home of the intended victim (Chesterton, 1972). Despite these precautions the murderer manages to enter the house unseen and carries out his homicidal plan. Each of the four men sent to guard the house denies seeing the murderer come and go. At the conclusion of the story, it becomes clear that the killer had been "invisible" to these men because he was the *postman*. The story illustrates how the same mind set that helps to conveniently arrange our world of experience can also cause blindness to unanticipated findings.

The clinical setting in which we practice, our typical clientele, the consensus of viewpoint sometimes adopted by clinicians who work together— all these factors fashion a context that can distort clinical observations. This effect was dramatically illustrated in a now-famous research study involving eight "pseudo-patients" admitted to one of twelve different mental treatment facilities (Rosenhan, 1973). The eight individuals who volunteered for this study included a graduate student, a housewife, a painter, three psychologists, a psychiatrist, and a pediatrician, none of whom had had any history of psychiatric problems. Individually, they presented themselves to treatment facilities with a standard complaint: "I have been hearing voices. They go empty, hollow, thud." Real names and occupations were not given; otherwise, the pseudo-patients were truthful in reporting their lives. All of them were admitted for treatment; and, all but one received a diagnosis of schizophrenia.

The research protocol prohibited these individuals from giving fictitious complaints *subsequent* to their hospital admission; in fact, they were required to speak of their admitting problem as though it were a thing of the past. This seemed to have little bearing on the length of their hospitalizations. They were retained for periods ranging from 7 to 52 days, with an overall average of 19 days. During the course of these various hospitalizations, collectively they received a total of 2,100 pills, which in most instances they managed to dispose of without detection. Upon discharge all were diagnosed as schizophrenic in remission.

The most telling finding of this study came out during follow-up interviews. Professional staff and patients were questioned about suspicions they might have had concerning the real identities of the pseudo-patients. Whereas none of the professionals indicated any suspicion, several patients related how they had guessed that these were not actual patients. The designer of the study commented: "The hospital itself imposes a special environment in which the meanings of behavior can easily be misunderstood" (Rosenhan, 1973).

Psychological masquerade is no respector of persons.

In the late 1930s the great American composer, George Gershwin began to suffer bouts of fatigue. This was soon followed by pounding headaches and a change in his personality. Friends found Gershwin moody and overly critical of others. But it all seemed understandable given the mounting stress in his life. After early and notable musical successes, he had made a film in Hollywood, "Shall We Dance," which had gotten less than rave reviews. Additionally, Gershwin and his brother, Ira, had agreed to work on a pet project of Samuel Goldwyn's known as the "Goldwyn Follies," a three-hour song and dance extravaganza. Gershwin found the project distasteful and didn't like having to cater to the primadonna whims of its producer.

About the same time, Gershwin found himself falling in love with a woman considerably younger than himself. He began to contemplate marriage. It all added up to considerable stress in his life. His friends thought (as he did) that it was just a little too much for him, his headaches and moodiness the resulting outcome.

The symptoms progressively worsened. Finally, Gershwin admitted himself to the Cedars of Lebanon Hospital in Los Angeles. For 26 days he was subjected to extensive testing by numerous specialists. Despite this exhaustive medical workup, he was discharged with the notation that it was "most likely hysteria."

At home Gershwin began to find light painful to his eyes (photophobia). He had to draw the blinds to keep out the sunlight. He became unsteady on his feet. Still friends and acquaintances persisted in their belief that it was all in George's mind. On one occasion he fell while walking along a sidewalk. One of the women accompanying him was heard to comment, "Leave him there. All he wants is attention."

Ira persisted in referring to the problem as a "nervous disorder." Gershwin continued to deteriorate. His headaches were unrelenting. He began to have trouble holding on to things. Finally, he was readmitted to the hospital and within a few days fell into a coma. An X-ray showed a mass compressing the right ventricle of the brain. At surgery it was first felt that the problem was a benign brain cyst, but the elation quickly faded when a highly malignant glioblastoma was found just underneath the cyst. The tumor was inoperable. Gershwin died the following day at the age of 39. (Jablonski, 1987)

Our increasing sophistication about psychosomatic stress reactions sets the stage for misinterpreting psychological masquerade. No one is immune.

As mental health professionals our clinical orientation must be "porous" enough to allow the registering of unexpected clues suggestive of organic mental disorders. We must be able to sift through the obvious in order to view the hidden. Our clinical task requires that we resist attending only to those items of information that conform to our favorite clinical explanations. Given that psychiatric symptoms are frequently best explained psychologically, we continually run the risk of being lulled into an insensitivity to organic mental disorders. The objective of this book is to render the reader more resistant to this clinical mistake.

BRIEF PREVIEW

In the following chapter we will consider the design of the nervous system, with emphasis on the structural basis of organic mental disorders.

Chapter 3 presents several clinical misconceptions that create blind spots for the clinician and predispose to errors in recognizing psychological masquerade.

Chapters 4 and 5 discuss basic guidelines for recognizing masquerading conditions. The approach takes brain syndrome as a starting point and adds other common clues.

In Chapter 6 a practical method is outlined for integrating a search for psychological masquerade into the clinical interview.

Four masqueraders are reviewed in Chapter 7, four kinds of organic disorders frequently misconstrued as psychological reactions: brain tumors, epilepsy, endocrine disorders, and AIDS.

Chapter 8 considers organic mental disorders induced by drugs, (including medications and alcohol). Chemical substances taken into the body are the number one cause of organic mental disorders.

The topic of somatization is taken up in Chapter 9 as a means of alerting the reader to findings that are *inconsistent* with a psychosomatic explanation of physical symptoms. The idea that physical symptoms can be manifestations of psychological conflicts can be too loosely applied as a clinical hypothesis, sometimes with tragic results.

Chapter 10 focuses on psychological masquerade in children and the elderly.

A brief summary of the major points of the book is provided in Chapter 11, as well as a self-test section of clinical cases for the reader's consideration.

Finally, there is an annotated bibliography, containing selected references relevant to psychological masquerade.

REFERENCES

Abercrombie, J. (1960). *The anatomy of judgement.* New York: Basic Books.

Chesterton, G. K. (1972). *Selected stories.* London: Kingsley Amis.

Hall, R., Popkin, M., DeVaul, R. A., Faillace, L., & Stickney, S. (1978). Physical illness presenting as psychiatric disease. *Archives of General Psychiatry, 35,* 1315–1320.

Hall, R., Gardner, E., Stickney, S., LeCann, A., & Popkin, M. (1980). Physical illness manifesting as psychiatric disease II: Analysis of a state hospital inpatient population. *Archives of General Psychiatry, 36,* 414–419.

Hofling, C. (1968). *Textbook of psychiatry for medical practice* (2nd ed.). Philadelphia: J. B. Lippincott.

Jablonski, E. (1987). *Gershwin.* New York: Doubleday.

Koran, L., Sox, H., Marton, K., Moltzen, S., Kraemer, H., Kelsey, T., Levin, L., Imai, K., Rose, T., & Chandra, S. (1989). Medical evaluation of psychiatric patients: I. Results in a state mental health system. *Archives of General Psychiatry, 46,* 733–740, 1989.

Koranyi, E. (1979). Morbidity and rate of undiagnosed physical illnesses in a psychiatric clinic population. *Archives of General Psychiatry, 36,* 414–419.

Rosenhan, D. (1973). On being sane in insane places. *Science, 179,* 250–258.

Rubert, S., & Remington, F. (1962). Why patients with brain tumors come to a psychiatric hospital: A 30-year survey. *American Journal of Psychiatry, 119,* 256–257.

Slater, E. (1965). Diagnosis of "hysteria." *British Medical Journal, 1,* 1395–1399.

Spark, R., White, R., & Connolly, R. B. (1980). Impotence is not always psychogenic. *JAMA, 243,* 750–755.

Tissenbaum, M., Harter, H. & Friedman, A. (1951). Organic neurological syndrome diagnosed as functional disorders. *JAMA, 147,* 1519–1521.

Chapter 2

Design of the Nervous System

Man seems to be a rickety poor sort of thing . . . A machine that was as unreliable as he is would have no market. —Mark Twain

The human nervous system is a complex communications network. Messages from the outside world are picked up by specialized sensory detectors in the form of light (vision), chemical reactions (taste, smell) and mechanical stimulation (touch, vibration, sound). They are then transmitted over peripheral channels into a central processing area where they are analyzed and interpreted in relation to other information, past and present. Outgoing messages are generated and, in turn, translated into various responses: muscle action, speech, emotional response, glandular activity, contemplation, and many others. Through this arrangement, the nervous system is able to maintain contact with the outside world as well as with the other systems of the human body on which it is vitally dependent. This communication network enables the nervous system to plan and direct the essential human activities of protection, maintenance, growth, and creation.

Skill in clinical assessment is enhanced by a working knowledge of the design of the nervous system. This does not necessitate a detailed understanding of neurophysiology or neuroanatomy, but rather a basic grasp of the common "break points." This chapter highlights those aspects of the nervous system that carry the greatest potential for going awry and giving rise to organic mental disorder.

THE BRAIN AND ITS HOUSING

Brain substance is not very durable. It resembles a firm gelatin. A rigid, bony covering—the skull and spinal vertebrae—and three layers of coverings that separate the brain from its stone-like housing provide protection. In addition the brain and spinal cord are further insulated by cerebrospinal fluid contained within the surrounding membranous layers.

This arrangement, however, is not invincible. While protecting against external trauma to the brain, this rigid casing—incapable of expansion—predisposes the brain to other dangers. If fluid collects within the brain (as sometimes occurs with infection or bleeding) or if tumorous growth develops, there is no "give" in the brain's rigid housing. The only outcome is inward encroachment on brain substance, often producing prominent psychiatric symptoms.

Another potential problem relates to the fluid in which the brain is suspended. Cerebrospinal fluid not only surrounds the brain and spinal cord, it also flows through the brain by way of a series of small canals known as ventricles. These passageways are relatively narrow and can be obstructed by tumorous growth, swelling, or hemorrhage. The destructive outcome is similar to the effect of damming a river. Increased pressure builds behind the obstruction. The growing pressure cannot be dissipated outward because of the rigid housing. Instead, the brain substance is "pressured" into dysfunction or even death. In newborn infants—because the skull has not yet ossified into bone—blockage of one of these fluid channels in the brain produces an outward enlargement of the cartilaginous skull, resulting in the enormous head size seen in hydrocephalus. Eventually, however, the limits of accommodation are reached, and the rising intracranial pressure is transmitted inward. Severe mental retardation is the outcome.

The soft coverings (meninges) of the brain while providing a degree of protection can become infected, giving rise to a condition known as meningitis. Typically manifested by stiff neck and headache, meningitis can also cause confusion, bizarre behavior, or even personality changes. In certain cases the invading infectious agents—particularly viruses—attack the brain itself, causing encephalitis. In effect, billions of nerve cells are invaded by an outside agent which consumes the brain's nutrients and otherwise interferes with its functioning. The resulting clinical picture ranges from subtle headache and fatigue to gross aberrations in thinking, sensing, moving, and behaving. Sometimes behavioral changes are the most prominent manifestation.

MESSAGE TRANSMISSION

The basic unit of the human nervous system is the neuron. Billions of these microscopic cells are intricately woven into a vast communication network.

Each neuron is composed of three elements: a cell body, an axon, and dendrites. Through a chemical language, messages are conveyed from one neuron to another.

Neurons do not make actual physical contact. They are microscopically separated by spaces known as synapses. The "gap" requires a special means of transmitting messages from one neuron to another in the form of chemical vehicles called neurotransmitters (Omenn, 1976). These chemical messengers are released at the end of one neuron. Through chemical diffusion, the transmitter reaches the other side and communicates its message, either positive or negative (excitatory or inhibitory), to a neuroreceptor on the adjacent neuron. The state of the nervous system is the ongoing summation of these positive and negative messages across billions of neurons. Out of this neurochemical process, human experience emerges.

Several different chemical messengers convey messages to different parts of the brain. Some are highly concentrated in certain brain sites, while others are found throughout the nervous system. A common potential problem shared by all neurotransmitters is saturation. Once a neurotransmitter has been released from one neuron and has communicated its message to an adjacent neuron, the chemical messenger must be destroyed in order to open up the communicative channel. In other words, the signal that has been given previously must be turned off before a new message can be sent. This message-erasing is also accomplished chemically. Communication within the nervous system is dependent on neurotransmitters and their receptors, the chemicals that erase them and the relative proportions of neurotransmitters to one another and to the erasing chemicals.

What is the clinical significance of this chemical brain language? Neurotransmitters and their erasers are similar to a variety of drugs, both medicinal and nonmedicinal. This fact sets the stage for the striking behavioral changes that drugs are capable of inducing. Drugs can send inappropriate messages as a result of chemical "jamming." Drugs, including medications, cause mental disturbances by upsetting the chemical balance essential to normal brain communication. (We will consider this problem at greater length in a later chapter on drug-induced mental disorders.)

Neurons are wrapped in supportive sheaths made of myelin. Certain diseases selectively compromise these protective coverings and by doing so cause an electrical "short-circuiting." This is the problem in the disease known as multiple sclerosis. Demyelinization occurs episodically in patches scattered across the nervous system, the exact location determining the nature of the symptoms.

After 24 hours of nonstop activity, a 34-year-old secretary was arrested for stealing a motorbike. The evening before, she had gone to her employer's home, assaulted his son, and left with his motorcycle. As far as anyone could surmise, there had been no precipitating circumstance.

After initial observation, the woman was sent to a hospital. She was overly suspicious and spoke in a rapid, rhythmic speech pattern that at times evolved into clang associations. She was grandiose in her ideas and sexually provocative. Her concentration was poor, and she had little insight into her problem. She was, however, alert and fully oriented, and all other aspects of her neurological examination were normal.

There was a past history, one year earlier, of sudden blindness in the left eye associated with changes in sensation in her left leg. These symptoms rapidly cleared without any residual. Four weeks later, she was hospitalized for a prolonged spending spree. She had been overactive, talking rapidly and inappropriately told her boss he didn't know his job. She insisted that the firm would be better off if he put her in charge of all investments.

Based on her earlier episode of sudden, temporary, left-eye blindness combined with the results of a lumbar puncture showing lymphocytes in the cerebrospinal fluid, a diagnosis of multiple sclerosis was made. The patient's "manic attack" was presumed to be an expression of this demyelinating disease. She was treated with ten days of haloperidol and lithium.

After a gradual recovery, she returned to work and did well on lithium until her second attack a year later leading to her arrest for stealing a motorbike. (Kwentus, Hart, Calabrese, & HeKnati, 1986)

BRAIN SPECIALIZATION

Areas of specialization are scattered throughout the brain. They coordinate brain activities which when disturbed produce readily identifiable neurological problems. Other areas, however, do not directly affect motor movement or sensation; rather, they play vital roles in interpretation, integration, and subjective response. Deficits in these associative areas are often manifest as cognitive, behavioral or emotional changes rather than paralysis or loss of sensation.

The following brief descriptions focus on certain specialized areas which when disordered are prone to cause psychological masquerade.

Frontal Lobes

The frontal lobes are the most recently evolved part of the human brain. As the name implies, this area is located in the front part of the skull (bilaterally), representing approximately 50% of the brain's total surface area. A large part of the frontal lobes is not involved in motor movement and sensation—thus its characterization as a relatively "silent area." For this reason, it is quite possible for frontal lobe disease to progress for lengthy periods of time without the appearance of obvious neurological symptoms. The earliest signs may be subtle changes in thought, mood, behavior, and personality (Heilman, 1979).

The frontal area is involved in abstract thinking and logical problem solving. It is crucial to a person's ability to understand symbols and to perceive commonalities. For example, a person with frontal lobe disease may not comprehend that a plum, an orange, and an apple are three different kinds of fruit; instead, the person may be locked into the *shape* they share—round.

Common sense is also often compromised in frontal lobe disease. The person may be unable to answer simple hypothetical questions such as, what should be done if he should lose his house keys or if he should come across a stamped and addressed letter lying on the street. Similarly, simple math problems may prove highly difficult.

Impulse control is another important frontal-lobe activity. It is as though this part of the brain watches over primitive urges, ensuring that they are translated into more acceptable expressions. When impulse control is compromised, personal self care often deteriorates, and sexual and aggressive behaviors emerge that conflict with commonly accepted social mores.

The frontal lobes also influence motivation. Depending on the precise location, frontal lobe disorders can produce a restriction of motivation to the point of apathy; or in the other direction, a shift toward impulsive, manic behavior. The apathetic, unmotivated person withdraws from activities and loses the capacity for pleasure and humor. This can be mistaken for psychological depression. On occasion, frontal-lobe dysfunction becomes so severe that the person is immobilized, unable to initiate speech, a condition which resembles catatonic schizophrenia.

The opposite clinical picture of overactivity can be misconstrued as bipolar disorder. The person appears maniacal, driven, and unable to concentrate. He may relate in a sociopathic manner without regard for the feelings or welfare of others (even close friends).

Despite the relatively "silent" nature of the frontal lobes, certain changes in motor control and sensory experience are sometimes seen in advanced stages of disease. Due to connections with other parts of the brain, disturbances in walking characterized by a gradual decrease in the size of the steps and a deterioration in balance can develop. Bladder dysfunction, starting with a recurrent sense of urgency and progressing to complete loss of control, is also observed. Urinary incontinence should never be ignored in persons with mental problems!

Finally, as a result of the anatomical juxtaposition of the optic and olfactory nerves to the underside of the frontal lobes, disturbances in vision or a diminished sense of smell may accompany progressive frontal disease before other symptoms appear.

Temporal Lobes

The way we perceive the world is critically dependent on the temporal lobes. This middle portion of the brain integrates the tremendous variety of sensations received by the brain; thus, it is not surprising that temporal lobe disorders are frequently associated with gross perceptional distortions (Benson & Geschwind, 1975). Hallucinations such as unpleasant odors, strange visual imagery, or even the sound of distant music are sometimes experienced, as are distortions of an illusionary nature: everything suddenly growing large or suddenly shrinks; new surroundings abruptly seem familiar or well-known settings defy recognition. Such perceptual distortions can be easily mislabeled as "schizophrenic" or "hysterical."

On the dominant side of the brain (the left side in the vast majority of persons), a language area is located at the margin of the temporal and parietal lobes. This area is essential to the understanding and use of spoken and written language. Temporal lobe disorders which give rise to language aberrations suggest the rambling, incoherent verbal productions seen in psychosis. Actually they are manifestations of a condition known as aphasia. (More about this later.)

At their inner margins, the temporal lobes merge into the rest of the limbic system and have extensive connections with this ancient brain, the seat of primitive emotions. Consequently, temporal lobe disorders may cause the unprovoked release of powerful emotions, such as panic, rage, or hypersexuality.

After two years of "panic attack," a 69-year-old school teacher sought psychiatric treatment. She related a history of unprovoked anxiety that would suddenly sweep over her. In addition she found herself becoming depressed and crying. Antidepressant medication was prescribed (maprotiline, 50–75 mg/day). Within a few months, her depression was much improved; but the panic attacks persisted and she started having other symptoms. For brief moments, she would sense that things were unreal. This progressed to instances of perceiving persons' faces change in size.

After a few more months, these bizarre visual experiences stopped, but she continued to have panic attacks, particularly in the afternoons. Then abruptly, there was a new development. While talking with her sister, she began to stare, unresponsively, at the wall. For ten minutes she seemed completely unaware. Afterward she was able to talk but appeared confused and was unable to answer simple questions. She could not recall her address or her husband's work telephone number.

Upon being taken to an emergency room, she had a second staring attack during which she had a terrified look. and exhibited strange movements of her lips. A CAT scan revealed a right, temporal lobe meningioma, (confirmed by carotid angiograms). The tumor was removed surgically, and the patient was started on antiseizure medication along with an antidepressant. Eight months later she had had no more "spells." (Ghadirian, Gowthier, & Bertrand, 1986)

Associative Cortical Areas

Located as islands scattered through the brain are areas essential to object recognition and to understanding how to execute specific movements. Disruptions in these associative areas produce a variety of bewildering symptoms. Failure to grasp the significance of various objects (in the absence of any disturbance in the sensory pathways themselves) is called agnosia. The person will be unable to recognize familiar objects. To an outside observer, this bewildering deficit in recognition may appear bizarre if not psychotic.

The neurologist, Oliver Sacks, in his intriguing book, *The Man Who Mistook His Wife For A Hat*, describes a music instructor who became unable to recognize faces (Sacks, 1985). When students would arrive for their lessons, Dr. P. would not know who it was until they spoke. The voices he recognized; but the faces were foreign. In addition (although Dr. P. failed to recognize familiar faces) he would often visualize them when there were none to be seen. On the street, reminiscent of the famous Mr. Magoo character, he would pat the heads of water hydrants and parking meters, mistaking them for the heads of children.

Inside, things were not much better. He would amiably speak to the carved knobs on the furniture and became perplexed when they failed to answer.

At first these odd mistakes were laughed off. The problem, whatever it was, did not detract from Dr. P's dazzling musical ability. He did not feel ill; in fact, he seemed to be in perfect health. It was three years later, after the onset of diabetes, that Dr. P's strange affliction was finally diagnosed.

Knowing that diabetes could affect his eyes, Dr. P. consulted an ophthalmologist. After a careful history and eye examination, he was told there was nothing wrong with his eyes, but that the visual part of his brain was not working correctly. After being referred to a neurologist. Dr. P. was found to suffer from a degenerative process of the visual associative area. He lived several more years and continued teaching music to the very end.

A rare form of agnosia known as *anosognosia* leaves a person unaware of one side of his body, so that even when he is shown his own leg, he will adamantly deny it.

> A young man was admitted to the hospital for medical tests. On examination, his doctor had found what he described as a "lazy leg." The patient felt fine, but at the conclusion of the first day of tests, he was tired and fell asleep in his room. When he awakened, he felt strangely apprehensive and suddenly flung himself onto the floor of his hospital room.
>
> When discovered by a medical student, he related that he had found "someone's leg" in his bed, a severed leg, he had thought to himself, placed beside him while he was sleeping. He was simultaneously amazed and disgusted. When he felt the limb, it was cold and "peculiar." Being that it was New Year's Eve, he convinced himself that it was all part of a sick joke played by a drunken nurse. Angry, but relieved, he proceeded to hurl the disgusting limb onto the floor. Unfortunately, much to his dismay, it was attached to him! This is how he came to be laying in the middle of the floor holding onto his left leg.
>
> The man was unable to accept his situation. Instead, he proceeded to ragefully punch the appendage. Finally, he agreed to being placed back in bed. As this was done, he was asked where his own left leg was. He blanched pale. "I don't know," he said, "I have no idea." (Sacks, 1985)

This is a graphic example of the bizarre perceptual distortions seen with lesions involving the parietal lobes. Such experiences are not manifestations of psychosis; they are reflections of purietal-lobe brain dysfunction.

Apraxia, in contrast, is the inability (despite normal muscle strength and function) to carry out a desired action. Although fully aware of how he wants to move and what he wants to accomplish, the person cannot trans late this desire into action. Common tasks like dressing oneself defy solution. The person becomes perplexed and frustrated after repeated failures at carrying out routine tasks.

Difficulty copying simple geometric figures is another expression of apraxia. When the person attempts to copy triangles, squares or rectangles, the angles and lines are distorted. This constructional apraxia provides the basis for two clinical screening tests later described as the Draw-a-Clock and Copy-a-Three-Dimensional-Figure Tests.

Limbic System

From an evolutionary perspective, the limbic system is a much older brain than the cerebral cortex. It is the center of activities upon which individual and species survival depend (MacLean, 1964). One researcher has summarized these functions as the "four F's of the limbic system": feeding, fighting, fleeing, and the "undertaking of mating activity" (MacLean, 1958). Given its vital nature, it is not surprising that the limbic area is the initiator of powerful and primitive emotions like rage and terror. These feelings, as well as sexual urges, have been elicited by electrical brain stimulation. Dramatic mood changes, sometimes of psychotic proportion, have followed this kind of limbic surgical arousal. Normally, limbic impulses are modulated by higher cortical centers, but in various disease states, their expression goes unchecked.

In a famous research study on monkeys, the bilateral removal of portions of the limbic brain led to a bizarre constellation of behavioral changes (Kluver & Bucy, 1937). The animals became extremely docile, and they no longer experienced fear, as illustrated by their casually playing with snakes that previously had terrified them. In addition they engaged in indiscriminate sexual behavior and were observed to compulsively chew, lick, suck, and swallow.

Such studies convincingly demonstrate the unusual behavior that can arise from the limbic system. It is little wonder that destructive or irritative limbic diseases are frequently mistaken for emotional reactions. When it invades the nervous system, the herpes simplex virus preferentially attacks the limbic brain, resulting in an encephalitis characterized by striking emotional and behavioral changes. The following case history illustrates how easily this condition can be mistaken for a psychological problem, particularly when stressful interpersonal events occur simultaneously.

A 30-year-old-divorced woman was accompanied by her mother to the hospital. She was unable to relate a coherent history. "I'm crazy—maybe I have been crazy all my life," she said. She also expressed the feeling that she had been "living in a dream" and that things had seemed "unreal" for the past several weeks. The woman's mother described her as having been despondent and agitated. She had had a poor appetite and experienced difficulty falling asleep. In a two-week period she had lost 10 pounds and had become progressively more disorganized and confused.

Further history revealed that she had had a serious love affair with her employer, whom she had fully expected to marry after he was free from his wife. Shortly before her symptoms appeared, the man had taken his wife and family on an expensive vacation to the "island paradise" where the patient had anticipated moving with him when they were married. Her mother commented, "She acted like her dreams were shattered."

In the hospital the woman appeared frightened. Many of her answers to questions, particularly those regarding where she was and the time of day, were flippant, circumstantial, or inappropriate. At times her speech was incoherent, but no obvious hallucinations or delusional thinking were observed.

Her neurological examination was normal, as were her vital signs, with the exception of a slightly evalated pulse rate of 104. All admission laboratory work was normal. The provisional diagnosis was acute schizophreniform episode, precipitated by stress in her personal life.

Despite tranquilizer medication, the woman's condition worsened. She became mute and suffered obvious neurological deficits, including altered speech and leg paralysis. A diagnosis of herpes simplex encephalitis was finally made on the basis of a marked rise in antibodies to the herpes virus.

The patient eventually recovered, but at a follow-up visit one year later she still had some difficulty walking. (Wilson, 1976)

Autonomic Nervous System (ANS)

This part of the nervous system carries out automatic functions essential to body maintenance and coping with stress. Arising deep within the brain in the hypothalamus, the ANS divides into two segments: the sympathetic and the parasympathetic. The parasympathetic division initiates changes conducive to body maintenance and repair. Overall, it produces a general calming effect. The heart rate slows and the blood pressure drops. Blood is diverted from the muscles to the gastrointestinal tract as a means of promoting the absorption of nutrients. The pupils are constricted; the body temperature is slightly lowered. Energy is conserved.

In contrast, the sympathetic division readies the body for emergency response. Heart rate increases and blood pressure rises. Blood is selectively directed to the muscles, in preparation for action. The pupils are dilated; body temperature rises, and sweating ensues. Energy is expended in preparation for action. The body is placed on alert.

The two divisions of the ANS utilize different chemical communicators (neurotransmitters) which various drugs can enhance or block. ANS manifestations, easily observed by the alert clinician, often provide valuable clues to drug intoxication. For example, widely dilated pupils are seen when a person has used a stimulant such as cocaine. The same finding is seen when the parasympathetic division has been suppressed by an anticholinergic drug.

The ANS controls the body's vital signs (respiration, heart rate, blood pressure, and temperature). Sustained alterations in these measures are important clues to organic disease.

Basal Ganglia

Located in the mid-brain, the basal ganglia are complexes of neurons crucial to coordinated movement. As with the ANS, the functions of the basal ganglia depend on a proper neurotransmitter balance. When there is an excess of acetylcholine, a pervasive stiffness and rigidity results. An excess of dopamine leads to twitching and jerking. A balance between these two substances is essential to normal movement.

This same neurotransmitter balance is also essential to higher brain functioning having to do with consciousness and other complex human behavior. Treatment with psychoactive medications presumably improves the disturbed ratio of brain neurotransmitters; but, whereas a proper balance may be restored at higher cortical levels (thereby ameliorating the symptoms of psychosis) simultaneously an imbalance may be precipitated within the basal ganglia, creating disturbances of movement such as parkinsonian symptoms—stiffness, muscle spasms, and tremor—common side effects of most neuroleptic medications.

Several neurological disorders of movement characteristically include mental and emotional changes that sometimes are the initial manifestation of what will eventually become a full-blown neurological disorder. Huntington's chorea is a relentlessly progressive, degenerative neurological disease, affecting the basal ganglia and the cerebral cortex. It is characterized by explosive, involuntary writhing with muscle jerks and twitches and declining mental ability. Antisocial behavior, poor impulse control, hypersexuality, and frank psychosis are often present. These psychological changes may overshadow the abnormalities of movement and in certain cases are the first manifestations, emerging years before other neurological deficits.

> After a period of adolescent delinquency involving theft, drunkenness, and assault, a young man, aged 22, experienced the gradual onset of unexplained physical awkwardness. In a short while he also began to have strange facial grimacing and jerky movements in his arms which caused a menacing appearance.
>
> At 24 he married. Later, his wife would relate how he was extremely demanding, particularly sexually, insisting on intercourse frequently at inconvenient times and in inappropirate situations. If denied, he would become vindictive, if not actually violent.
>
> Three years after the marriage the man was commited to a criminal asylum after a vicious attack on his wife. By this time there was also an extensive history of brutality toward his children. His condition was diagnosed as psychopathic personality.
>
> Further investigation, however, revealed that the patient's mother had died at age 42 of Huntington's chorea. A thorough neurological evaluation confirmed that the patient was suffering the same fate. He had severe unsteadiness in walking, and his arms and legs flung wildly about. His speech was slurred, and he had a serious memory problem.
>
> The man's condition progressed until at the age of 32 he died of bronchopneumonia. (Dewhurst, 1970)

The integrity of the basal ganglia and psychological well-being (for reasons not completely understood) are closely tied together. All mental health professionals should be sensitized to the association of organic mental disorders and abnormalities of movement.

THE SUPPORTING CAST

Unlike simple life forms that carry out all life activities within a single cell, the human animal is highly specialized and requires the integrated performance of many different organ systems to conduct its routine, day-to-day business of living. As highly evolved organisms far from our ancient beginnings, humans are confronted with the complex task of maintaining a stable internal environment reminiscent of the primordial sea (Simeons, 1960). Slight variations in body temperature, oxygen availability, or salt concentration become life-threatening. Levels of various chemicals in the body must remain within a narrow range lest vital processes begin to fail. Waste products created from life-sustaining energy consumption must be eliminated regularly if death due to "internal pollution" is to be avoided.

The brain directs this complicated array of life-support processes; but, like most bosses, it is dependent on the activities of its subordinates. When members of the supporting cast fail, problems in brain functioning are not far behind. The emergence of psychiatric symptoms in a person with known medical disease should always alert the clinician to the possibility of brain disturbance secondary to a failing support system. This is why individuals with chronic diseases are particularly susceptible to psychological masquerade. Secondary brain problems are often more subtle in their presentations than are primary diseases of the nervous system. *Secondary brain failure* is an important concept for the clinician to keep in mind.

Heart, Lungs, and Blood

The brain is vitally dependent on an uninterrupted supply of oxygen. Sudden loss of oxygen produces coma in less than 60 seconds and death within a matter of five–six minutes. For oxygen to reach the brain, the lungs must remove it from the air and transfer it to the blood. In turn the heart must maintain a continuous flow of oxygen-laden blood by uninterrupted pumping. Certain alterations in the rhythm of the heart can compromise its pumping effectiveness and rapidly lead to brain dysfunction, loss of consciousness, and death unless the problem is immediately corrected. Other arrhythmias may not cause such drastic compromises in heart functioning but, instead, may produce subtle behavioral changes or subjective complaints. Consider the following case:

> A widowed woman, age 54, became guilt ridden and anxious following her husband's death. At times her heart would beat rapidly, and she would feel tense and fearful. The woman's children attributed these changes to her having "taken up" with her dead husband's former associate. She resisted this interpretation but eventually, with reluctance, agreed to see a psychiatrist.
>
> When the woman entered the psychiatrist's office, he noticed that she appeared unsteady on her feet and that her ankles were swollen. These observations, plus the patient's story of heart palpitations associated with a pervasive sense of dread, led to the diagnosis of paroxysmal atrial tachycardia, a heart condition characterized by sudden, explosive episodes of rapid heart action.
>
> Further investigation confirmed this diagnosis and also established the precise cause: a defective heart valve (mitral stenosis). After corrective surgery, the woman had no further attacks of anxiety or guilt, despite the continuation of her new relationship. (Shulman, 1977)

In addition to adequate heart pumping, the transporting of nutrient-rich blood to the brain requires that the "pipelines" be unobstructed. These arterial vessels running from the heart to the nervous system can become obstructed by clot formation, bleeding, or tumor encroachment. The resulting blockage produces what is commonly known as a stroke. The specific disability emanating from a stroke will depend on the precise location of the obstruction. If, for example, the blockage occurs in an artery supplying the motor cortex on the left side of the brain, the person will likely experience a weakness or complete paralysis of his right arm or leg or both. But not all strokes have such obvious physical consequences.

> Without any explanation, a 61-year-old banker failed to go to work one morning. Despite his wife's puzzled questioning, he gave no reason; furthermore, he never again returned to work or even so much as mentioned the bank where he had worked for years.
>
> The man was examined by several physicians who could find "nothing wrong." His wife, however, noted several other changes. Much of his charm and wit disappeared. Overnight, this once capable and dynamic man had been transformed into an apathetic, dull, and sexless person. He no longer assumed responsibilities, made decisions, or did any reading. He exhibited peculiar behaviors. On one occasion his wife watched him walk into a wall, as though he did not see it. Another time he suddenly fell to the floor and lost consciousness. Although he quickly recovered, for a moment, he was unable to speak clearly. Eventually he became confused and began to have difficulty shaving and dressing himself.

Several years later another medical appraisal led to the diagnosis of stroke. It was determined that this man had suffered a series of small strokes, accounting for the striking changes in his personality and the decline in his overall competence. (Alvarez, 1966)

Diseases which lead to complete oxygen deprivation are easily recognized as medical emergencies, but the clinician is often faced with more subtle presentations. When the brain's oxygen supply is slowly compromised, a diversity of psychiatric symptoms may arise, alone or in various combinations, including irritability, confusion, apathy, depression, suspiciousness, and bizarre behavior. Due to changes at the interface between the lungs and capillaries, chronic lung disease reduces the amount of oxygen diffusing into the bloodstream. Likewise, widespread tuberculosis or cancer of the lung can produce a similar problem.

Cancer of the lung is the most common cancer in American males, and its incidence among women is rapidly rising. Before lung cancer is medically detectable, mental disorder may result as an organic consequence. In some cases this is a reflection of the early spread of the disease to the brain; in others, the mental manifestations stem from a compromise in lung function due to the invading tumor cells. The lungs become unable to "breathe" properly, creating a relative deprivation of oxygen. The clinical result may be quite unlike that anticipated from lung disease.

The man was strong of body and mind, a bricklayer, 53 years of age. Although rarely given to drink, he was a heavy smoker, consuming 40 cigarettes a day. He was described by friends as full of nervous energy, restless, often worried over things, sometimes depressed, but never bad-tempered.

Over a six-month period, he changed. His appetite failed and he slept poorly. He appeared vacant at times. Gradually, he became less outgoing, and when he was with others, he was frequently quarrelsome.

On a holiday, he suddenly became excited, burst out of his house and ran across the field in the early morning hours, shouting that he had to go to work. He was reassured by his family and for several months there were no further occurrences. He then began to make strange demands on his wife to meet him in distant places. When she would arrive, he might not be there; or, if he did appear, he might wander off suddenly without explanation.

He became religiously preoccupied and eventually violent. On one occasion he locked his wife and one of his children in a room with himself and proceeded to read loudly from the Bible. Periodically, he called out to "Lord Jesus" and scribbled strange sayings on the walls. When the police arrived, he threw the Bible on the fire; and, then in front of the onlooking officers, he grabbed burning coals from the fireplace and rubbed them across his own face, sustaining burns about his forehead.

The man was taken to the local hospital and admitted to the psychiatric ward, where he was diagnosed as having paranoid schizophrenia. He improved enough to be discharged and returned to work, but shortly thereafter suffered a severe vacant attack and was readmitted to the hospital completely irrational, pacing up and down and talking nonsense.

His condition rapidly deteriorated and twelve days later he died. At autopsy the cause for his "paranoid schizophrenia" was found to be cancer of the lung. (Charaton & Brierly, 1956)

Heavy smokers are at risk for emphysema and chronic bronchitis as well as lung cancer. Unexplained "psychological symptoms" in this high-risk population necessitates a thorough evaluation of pulmonary function (as well as a close examination of the medications being used).

Gastrointestinal Tract

The brain and the gastrointestinal tract derive from related germ plasm. Perhaps this accounts, in part, for the close association between psychological stress and gastrointestinal dysfunction such as irritable bowel syndrome (spastic colon), ulcerative colitis, and ulcers of the stomach and duodenum.

The stomach, intestines, pancreas, liver, and gall bladder are essential to the proper digestion, absorption, and conversion of food into usable energy. When they become dysfunctional, psychological symptoms are often part of the clinical picture. For example, in certain conditions (ulcer, inflammation, drug effects), the stomach and intestines become sources of occult blood loss. As this slow hemorrhaging occurs, the person may develop symptoms of fatigue secondary to anemia. When he or she complains of having no energy, the clinician may mistakenly perceive this as symptomatic of depression.

The liver is the site of hundreds of enzymatic reactions. It plays an important role in maintaining proper blood sugar levels and is responsible for detoxifying the waste products of normal metabolism. When the liver fails, the brain is quick to suffer, as in severe cases of acute viral hepatitis or in end-stage hepatic failure associated with alcoholic cirrhosis. Lethargy and difficulty concentrating may progress to full-blown brain syndrome and psychosis.

The brain's energy supply is glucose. Its continuous availability is essential to normal brain functioning. Unlike other parts of the body, the brain cannot use other forms of caloric energy. Since it has no inherent supply, the brain is completely dependent on other organ systems to secure its energy.

Because the ingestion of glucose is periodic, a storage reservoir is necessary to ensure adequate glucose at all times. The liver serves as an important warehouse where glucose is stored as glycogen for future use. When blood glucose drops, glycogen is broken down and diffuses into the blood to become available to the rest of the body and, most importantly, to the brain which takes a disproportionate share. Conditions that impair the liver, make a person more vulnerable to becoming hypoglycemic with dramatic cognitive and behavioral changes.

> Against her will, a 69-year-old-black woman was brought to a psychiatric emergency service by the police.
>
> Agitated and inattentive, she was unable to give a coherent story. Her speech was rambling and loose. She was disoriented in time and space, insisting that she was in jail.
>
> On physical examination, her liver was enlarged 2 cm below the lower margin of her right rib cage. A serum glucose was drawn. The result showed an extremely low level. Upon receiving 50 ml of 50% glucose IV-push, the patient immediately became coherent and attentive.
>
> She gave a history of 40 years of alcohol abuse, cirrhosis of the liver and pancreatitis (eventually necessitating a 95% pancreatectomy) and adult-onset diabetes, necessitating the regular use of insulin. On the morning of her hospitalization, accidentally, she had taken too much insulin and this had caused her profound hypoglycemia. (Fishbain & Rotundo, 1988)

Endocrine System

Endocrine glands manufacture hormones that act as powerful chemical stimulants, influencing growth, metabolism, sex reproduction, and emergency responses. Endocrine disorders often produce mental and emotional changes. Fortunately, most of these conditions are rare. Not so, however, in the case of thyroid disorders. They are prominent on any listing of cases of psychological masquerade.

The thyroid controls the body's rate of metabolism. Excess thyroid hormone causes irritability and anxiety. In severe cases, mania and paranoid psychosis may result. Too little thyroid hormone, in contrast, produces the opposite clinical picture: lethargy and depression. In severe hypothyroidism, dementia with slow-onset brain syndrome is the outcome.

As we saw in the previous case, insulin plays an essential part in the regulation of blood glucose. It is manufactured in the pancreas, a small endocrine gland attached to the intestinal tract (duodenum). Destructive processes such as inflammation, tumors, and trauma can impair the ability of the pancreas to produce and secrete insulin; consequently, the blood sugar level becomes quite erratic: too low at times, too high at others.

Diabetes mellitus is a deficiency disease resulting from failure of the pancreas to produce adequate amounts of insulin. In its most severe form (Type I), diabetes develops early in a person's life and requires daily injections of insulin without which death occurs. Some individuals with Type I diabetes have major difficulty achieving a stable level of blood sugar; consequently, despite taking insulin injections, they may have wide swings in blood sugar with concomitant psychological changes. If the clinician has no prior knowledge of a diabetic condition, these manifestations can easily be misconstrued.

Even in less severe cases of diabetes (Type II), significant mental and emotional changes may occur. On the basis of extensive investigation, one researcher identified a high incidence of diabetic problems among psychiatric patients (Koranyi, 1979). A clinical account included in his report described a couple who seemed on the verge of divorce. They had a pattern of nightly quarreling. Marital therapy had been tried without any improvement in what was a rapidly deteriorating relationship. Eventually, a test that measures the body's reaction to a standard quantity of ingested sugar (5-hour Glucose Tolerance Test) was given. It showed that approximately 3 hours after a meal both the husband and wife had a significant drop in blood sugar, presumably due to the excessive release of insulin. This "after dinner hypoglycemia" was giving rise to the irritable, anxious, subjective feelings experienced by the quarreling couple. (In Chapter 7 we will further explore the gamut of psychiatric symptoms associated with endocrine disorders, particularly those involving the thyroid gland.)

Liver and Kidneys

As the human body consumes energy, it generates waste products that must be eliminated. Under normal circumstances, this task is ably handled by special pollution-control systems within the body of which the liver and kidneys are key elements. Although both of these organs have tremendous reserve potential, when diseased their limits can be reached, leading to the toxic accumulation of waste products. In a polluted environment, the brain begins to fail. If the pollution is slow in developing, initially, there may be only subtle changes. The person becomes inattentive, apathetic or withdrawn. As the condition progresses, more serious alterations are likely: loss of the correct sense of time and place, failing memory for recent events, and the inability to solve simple problems. If the pollution goes unchecked, the person completely loses contact with reality experiencing delusions and hallucinations, easily mistaken for functional psychosis.

The kidneys can be compromised by infection. They are also susceptible to damage from certain medications and toxic products such as heavy metals and industrial chemicals. They can be injured as the target organ of autoimmune reactions where the body's own immune cells attack the kidneys by mistake. Regardless of the cause, when the kidneys are seriously damaged, serious mental and emotional changes are likely to appear.

In this chapter we have reviewed certain aspects of the nervous system (and its supporting cast) that underlie the development of organic mental disorders. Now we are ready to consider the common clinical traps that lead to errors in distinguishing psychological problems from organic disorders.

REFERENCES

Alvarez, W. (1966). *Little strokes.* Philadelphia: J. B. Lippincott.

Benson, D. F., & Geschwind, N. (1975). Psychiatric conditions associated with focal lesions of the central nervous system. *American Handbook of Psychiatry, 4* 208–243.

Charaton, F. B., & Brierley, J. B. (1956). Mental disorder associated with primary lung carcinoma. *British Medical Journal, 2,* 765–768.

Dewhurst, K. (1970). Personality disorder in Huntington's disease. *Psychiatrica Clinica, 3,* 221–229.

Fishbain, D., & Rotundo, D. (1988). Frequency of hypoglycemic delirium in a psychiatric emergency service. *Psychosomatics, 29,* 346–348.

Ghadirian, A., Gowthier, S., & Bertrand, S. (1986). Anxiety attacks in a patient with a right temporal lobe meningioma. *Journal of Clinical Psychiatry, 47,* 270–271.

Heilman, K. (1979). Exploring the enigmas of frontal lobe dysfunction. *Geriatrics, December,* 81–87.

Kluver, H., & Bucy, P. C. (1937). Psychic blindness and other symptoms following bilateral temporal lobectomy in Rhesus monkeys. *American Journal of Physiology. 119,* 353–363.

Koranyi, E. (1979). Morbidity and rate of undiagnosed physical illnesses in a psychiatric clinic population. *Archives of General Psychiatry, 36,* 414–419.

Kwentus, J., Hart, R., Calabrese, V., & HeKnati, A. (1986). Mania as a symptom of multiple sclerosis. *Psychosomatics, 27,* 729–731.

MacLean, P. (1958). Contrasting functions of limbic and neocortical systems of the brain and their relevance to psychophysiological aspects of medicine. *American Journal of Medicine, 25,* 611–626.

MacLean, P. (1964). Man and his animal brains. *Modern Medicine, 3,* 95–106.

Omenn, G. (1976). Neurochemistry and behavior in man. *Western Journal of Medicine, 125,* 434–451.

Sacks, O. (1985). *The man who mistook his wife for a hat.* London: Duckworth.

Shulman, R. (1977). Psychogenic illness with physical manifestations and the other side of the coin. *Lancet, i,* 524–526.

Simeons, A. (1960). *Man's presumptuous brain.* London: Longmans.

Wilson, L. (1976). Viral encephalopathy mimicking functional psychosis. *American Journal of Psychiatry, 133,* 165–170.

Chapter 3

Clinical Traps

Even brute beasts and wandering birds do not fall into the same traps or nets twice.
—St. Jerome

If clinicians consistently avoid certain conceptual errors, the chances of detecting psychological masquerade are greatly improved.

In this chapter we will review four clinical traps:

- Mistaking symptoms for their cause
- Getting seduced by the story
- Equating psychosis with schizophrenia (or functional psychosis)
- Relying (unnecessarily) on limited information

MISTAKING SYMPTOMS FOR THEIR CAUSE

Labeling has a certain magical quality to it. As clinicians, we sometimes lull ourselves into a false sense of certainty by applying a clinical label. It is as though by naming the symptom, we will fully understand it. One author has called this proclivity the "Rumpelstiltskin Complex," after the wonderful fairy tale about a lady who, in order to save herself from the power of an evil, ugly little man, had to correctly guess his name, Rumpelstiltskin (Torrey, 1972). At one level this fairy tale describes our magical belief in the process of naming. Name it, understand it, control it!

But such magic is not always productive. Sometimes labeling leads us astray. This is particularly true of commonly used adjectives that incorrectly have come to imply psychological etiology—terms like anxious, depressed, paranoid, obsessive, catatonic, and manic. In actuality, these clinical adjectives signify nothing with respect to causation. Both organic and psychological problems give rise to these symptoms. The symptoms, themselves, cannot be trusted to differentiate organic mental disorders from psychological reactions.

Descriptive labeling does not provide causative understanding.

Paranoia

Our psychosocial development depends on the resolution of a series of fundamental life crises. The degree of success we experience in resolving one crisis powerfully influences our handling of subsequent crises. According to this perspective, the first and most important crisis concerns trust versus mistrust (Erikson, 1963). Although this developmental crisis may be more favorably resolved by some of us than others, for all of us it remains somewhat of an open question throughout our lives; so, it is not surprising that instances of irrational suspiciousness are experienced from time to time by a majority of people. Given half a chance, paranoia emerges, often under conditions of increased stress or incomplete information, or drug intoxication.

Being paranoid is characterized by a constellation of symptoms centering around unwarranted suspicion. While contradictory evidence is ignored, "facts"—even the most insignificant and irrelevant—are selectively collected to prove the person's suspicions. Feelings associated with paranoia are predictably those of fear and anxiety, as well as an obsessive concern with the objects of suspicion.

As paranoia intensifies, frequently a distinct belief emerges that there is a plot afoot to harm the individual, which in turn may lead to a growing conviction in one's own supernatural powers or cosmic importance. When paranoia reaches this stage, it becomes totally absorbing, capable of distorting all evidence and fashioning supporting proof out of the most irrelevant observations: It reaches psychotic intensity. The severely paranoid person is extremely cautious, reluctant to give information, often speaking in guarded fashion so as not to be overheard. Despite such precautions, the feeling of being trapped periodically surfaces. Panic may erupt and on occasion lead to acts of violence, presumably out of a perceived need for self-defense.

Clinicians often mistake paranoia for schizophrenia.

A young soldier, 26 years of age, abruptly became apprehensive and suspicious. He was obsessed with the idea that "the Nationals" were trying to kill him.

The soldier appeared extremely anxious. He was disoriented and exhibited a rapidly fluctuating paranoid fear. At its height, this fear was clearly delusional.

The soldier's thinking was disjointed. His body coordination was impaired and his eyes notably reddened.

Over the next few hours, the soldier's condition rapidly improved. Eventually, he was able to relate that, just prior to the onset of this frightening experience, he had smoked marijuana.

Two days later he returned to duty. There was no recurrence during a 3-month follow-up period. (Talbott & Teague, 1969)

The reader should note that the clinical clues to this toxic condition came not so much from observing the paranoid behavior, but rather from taking note of its sudden onset, combined with body incoordination, disorientation and a reddening of the eyes. Nothing about the paranoia per se was diagnostic of an organic condition.

Consider a second case.

Officials at a local airport anxiously requested the assistance of the state police when a married school teacher in his late forties created a threatening scene. He became combative and began to scream about "doctors trying to kill him" with poison pills that would lead to "death by dehydration." The man frantically maintained that it was essential he make contact with the CIA and the Food and Drug Administration to prevent this crime against himself.

Following admission to the psychiatric service of a general hospital, he appeared confused and was unable to give the correct month. He continued to express persecutory delusions.

Routine laboratory tests showed a severe water and chemical imbalance known as *water intoxication.* With restriction of fluids, the confusional state promptly cleared. The paranoid delusions persisted for a brief time, but completely resolved after treatment with an antipsychotic medication. (Rosenbaum, Tothman, & Murray, 1979)

Numerous cases of water intoxication causing dramatic behavioral alterations have been reported. In some instances this strange condition has been traced to the inappropriate production of a hormone in the body known as antidiuretic hormone (ADH). An excess of this hormone prevents the proper excretion of water and leads to a "flooding" of the body. Other cases result from excessive water drinking.

A subgroup of chronic psychiatric patients—particularly high among those who suffer from long-standing schizophrenia—drink large amounts of water. (Illowsky & Kirch, 1988) Some go on to develop water intoxication which in its most severe form can be life-threatening. One review of schizophrenic patients under the age of 53 found water intoxication accounting for 18.5% of hospital deaths in this group (Vieweg et al., 1985). Clinical recognition of water intoxication depends on linking these symptoms to a history of excessive water consumption or decreased urinary output. When neurological manifestations are present (such as headaches, blurred vision, seizures, or decreasing consciousness), the organic nature of water intoxication should be obvious. As with the man in the airport, however, other symptoms can be overshadowing. The person may become restless, irritable, manic, confused, paranoid.

Paranoid reactions are frequently encountered by the clinician. Their causative basis can be organic as well as psychological.

Depression

The term, "depression," means different things ranging from "the blues" to suicidal and psychotic melancholia. Depression describes a broad spectrum of symptomatogy, induced by a host of different factors.

Despite the highly popular clinical notion that depression results from failure to express anger or resentment (usually in relation to some form of personal loss), it is important to keep its multiple etiologies in mind. Many organic disorders are heralded by depressive changes prior to the emergence of physical symptoms. This occurs commonly in cases of cancer, endocrine diseases, degenerative diseases, and subclinical infections. Also, medications are a frequent cause of depression in patients being treated for other problems.

Clinicians should be careful not to overreach for personal loss as an explanation for depression. Few persons go for extended periods without setbacks—financial, social, occupational, romantic, or symbolic. Such losses are not invariably the cause of depression. Individuals who become depressed due to organic illness may also have a notable personal loss that is of little etiological consequence. Personal loss can be misleading clue in cases of organic conditions presenting as depression.

Regardless of its cause, the defining characteristics of depression are sadness, a diminished sense of self-worth, restricted initiative, and a reduced capacity for pleasure. Changes in appetite and sleeping habits may occur. For some, food no longer seems desirable and weight loss ensues; for others, depression leads to voracious eating and weight gain. Persons who are depressed may have trouble falling asleep, and even when sleep finally comes, it may not last for long. Atypically, the opposite symptoms may be experienced: excessive sleep which appears to provide temporary escapes from a painful depressed mood.

Usually, depression is accompanied by decreased activity. The person cannot seem to get going; a sense of tiredness pervades his or her life. In its extreme form, psychomotor retardation immobilizes the person, leading to poor self-care. In other cases agitation is prominent. The individual appears anxious, irritable, and is easily provoked. Even with agitated depression, however, the more characteristic expressions of depression are never far from the surface.

Severe depression is a frequent precursor of suicidal thoughts and delusional thinking (mood consistent) such as thoughts of rotting insides, possession by the devil, or personal guilt for all of the world's wrongs.

Clinical recognition of depression does not resolve the question of etiology.

A 29-year-old woman, a college graduate, was seen at a psychiatric clinic for what she described as depression. For several months she had felt "down" to the extent of considering that life might be an unnecessary burden. She would awaken early in the morning. After being unable to fall back to sleep, she would feel lethargic the following day. Even more disturbing to her, she experienced a growing alienation from her children and husband.

Depression ran in the woman's family. Her father had committed suicide, and her mother had suffered from an involutional depressive psychosis. The woman herself had been severely depressed on two previous occasions, once shortly after starting on birth control pills and again immediately following the birth of her second child.

Given this history of hormonal-related depression, she was advised to stop the "pill," and, simultaneously, was referred for outpatient psychotherapy for her current depressive symptoms. Over the next several weeks, her depression lifted and her relationship with her family improved.

Six months later the woman discussed contraception with a psychiatrist. He encouraged her to return to her gynecologist for an alternative birth control method. Instead, as a means of economizing, she resumed taking the birth control pills that she still had at home. Within one week she was severaly agitated and depressed and required admission to a state mental hospital. A schizoaffective reaction was diagnosed.

After her release she suffered yet another episode of severe depression, complicated by hallucinations and strong impulses to kill her children. This occurred when she was started on another birth control pill! Upon cessation of the pill, the symptoms promptly disappeared.

The woman was thoroughly instructed about the relationship between her mental episodes and the taking of oral contraceptives. At a follow-up visit, she reported no further symptoms. (Daley, Kane & Ewing, 1967)

Hormonal-related depression is not a rare condition, particularly in women with a family history of mood disturbances (manic or depressive). As in the preceding case, this form of depression can be precipitated by birth control pills, or by pregnancy or its termination. In some instances depression occurs monthly with a woman's menstrual period. Presumably, this premenstrual pattern is related to hormonal changes.

Although people with psychological depression sometimes exaggerate minor somatic aches and pains, *persistent* physical complaints should never be assumed to be psychological without appropriate medical evaluation. They suggest an underlying, organic disorder.

> A 60-year-old lawyer became obviously depressed. His energy and initiative steadily declined. Upon falling asleep at night, he would soon awaken. He had an extensive history of depressive episodes; some had been severe, requiring electroconvulsive therapy.
>
> Along with the advent of his current depression, he had suffered an unexplained bout of persistent diarrhea. It was this troublesome physical symptom that brought him to a physician who, upon reviewing the case, concluded that the diarrhea was simply a manifestation of his depression.
>
> He was referred, however, to a consulting psychiatrist who decided that further investigations were indicated. Results showed the patient had ulcerative colitis. He responded favorably to steroid medications and experienced a resolution of his depression. (Shulman, 1977)

In recent years evidence has accumulated that in certain cases mood disturbances are closely tied to the seasons. Seasonal affective disorder (SAD), is characterized by winter depression with increased sleepiness, fatigue, weight gain, and carbohydrate craving. During the spring and summer, there is a reversal of symptoms which may even progress to a manic state (Rosenthal et al., 1984).

Exposure to light seems to play a key role in this seasonal mood swing. When *phototherapy* is administered daily, the symptoms disappear.

Mania

In contrast to the lowered self-esteem, absence of pleasure, and sloweddown feeling seen in depression, manic behavior produces euphoria—unreasonably so—with a falsely inflated self-image and a tendency to be flighty and overactive. The person becomes obsessed with his own importance; fun and pleasure are pursued at any cost; and, delusional beliefs of omnipotence and grandiosity emerge. Characteristically, the manic person rarely sleeps and has a diminished appetite. If the episode continues for long, significant weight loss can result.

The euphoric and heightened activity, however, does not lead to improved performance. Work and family relationships typically are severely compromised during manic episodes.

Encountering someone with full-blown mania is a memorable experience. It is difficult to get a word into the conversation, and keeping up with the one-sided conversation is next to impossible as the person flits from one topic to another with, at best, a tenuous thread of coherence. The manic person can be quite entertaining; the humor is infectious, and the interviewer may find himself laughing despite considerable effort at maintaining composure. At the slightest hint of being ignored or resisted, however, the nonstop joking and laughter may abruptly be replaced by irritation or outright belligerence.

Although manic episodes are associated with bipolar disorder (a cyclical mood disorder that runs in families), this is not invariably the cause. The clinical literature contains many examples of mania resulting from many organic disorders, including influenza, brain tumors, complex partial seizures, metabolic imbalances, strokes, as well as various drug reactions (cocaine, caffeine, tricyclic antidepressants, and steroids).

> A 69-year-old, retired drawbridge operator (without previous psychiatric history) abruptly developed an inappropriate euphoria that progressed over a 5-week period into flagrant manic behavior. Having become intolerable to his exhausted family, he was admitted to a hospital.
>
> When interviewed, the man aggressively accused his physician of plotting against him. He demanded to call his lawyer so that he might bring suit against the hospital. His family described inflated self-confidence, hyperactive behavior, and diminished inhibitions.
>
> For eight years the patient had suffered from Parkinson's disease. Recently, he had started on a new medication, L-Dopa. He showed no improvement until a dosage of 3 grams a day was reached. At this point his Parkinsonian tremor and rigidity suddenly disappeared; and, simultaneously, a profound shift in mood occurred. This was when his manic behavior began.
>
> The patient was suffering from an organic psychosis induced by L-Dopa. With an adjustment in dosage, the symptoms subsided. (Ryback & Schwab, 1971)

L-Dopa has proven to be an effective treatment for Parkinson's disease. It is not, however, without side effects, manic behavior being one of them.

An unusually high incidence of mania has been reported in women with endometriosis, a condition caused by an overgrowth of the lining of the uterus. Typically, women with this condition have excessive pain during menstruation. Depression—not mania—would be expected, but, in a study of sixteen consecutive cases of endometriosis, ten women (62%) met DSM-III criteria for bipolar disorders. The researchers pointed out that abnormal levels of the same hormone have been implicated in both disorders (Lewis et al., 1987).

We tend to associate "having a stroke" with weakness, slurred speech, and difficulty walking. This is a misleading stereotype; not all strokes cause such obvious neurological deficits. Strokes have been known to present as manic behavior.

> When, finally, he was admitted, he spoke in a nonstop fashion, proclaiming that he was both Christ and Hare Krishna. Interspersed in an endless flow of loosely jointed ideas, he extended invitations for the staff to kiss his feet.
>
> The man was 61 years old. Over the course of a few days, he had undergone a marked change. He became wildly euphoric and tirelessly active. He stopped sleeping altogether. Religion preoccupied him. He proselytized on the streets trying to convert others to his newfound belief. All of this was completely out of character. At times he became irritable and even aggressive toward his aged mother.
>
> In the hospital he was judged to be fully oriented. Tests of language, calculation and abstraction were normal, but he did have difficulty recalling three objects after three minutes. Oddly, in a drawing he rendered, he showed almost complete neglect of the left side. This led to a neurological examination that established the loss of his left visual field and diminished sensations of pain, temperature, and vibration.
>
> On the basis of these findings, the man was judged to have suffered a right thalamic stroke, too small to be seen on CT scan. The manic symptoms responded well to short-term lithium treatment; but, although the neurological deficits improved, he was left with some residual deficit. (Cummings & Mendez, 1984)

Anxiety

Anxiety is the disquieting sense of being threatened or of losing control. It may erupt episodically in the form of attacks or be sustained over long periods of time. Unlike fear, anxiety often stems from no clearly identifiable threat. The anxious person becomes preoccupied with his condition, thereby producing further anxiety. Even in its milder versions, anxiety usually includes a foreboding sense of the future. Anxiety and depression often fuse as emotional experiences and may be difficult to distinguish clinically.

Physical expressions of anxiety are usually prominent: tremulousness, a worried look, increased perspiration, and muscle tension, particularly in the muscles of the face, neck, and jaw. The muscle tension characteristically involves the muscles of the spine, giving the person a rigid appearance. It is not surprising that anxiety is often associated with increased body aches and pains, particularly headache and back discomfort.

Anxiety can be manifest behaviorally as increased restlessness. The person fidgets or paces. Tension-binding habits like smoking, drinking, and other drug use increase. Sexual acting out may provide temporary comfort.

Organic conditions that stimulate the sympathetic nervous system are easily mistaken for anxiety disorder. Long before they are diagnosed, physical diseases may be experienced by the person as anxiety, sometimes with a sense of impending doom. As discussed in Chapter 7, hyperthyroidism and hypoglycemia typically produce the outward appearance of anxiety.

In the following case, organic anxiety was incorrectly interpreted as a psychiatric problem.

> An unmarried piano teacher, 39 years of age, was chronically nervous. Fifteen years earlier he had been accused by one of his pupils of sexual advances. The accusation led to a court case. The teacher was eventually acquitted, but the experience was a severe emotional trauma that left him extremely nervous.
>
> Ten years later the man became noticeably more anxious and suffered daily bouts of diarrhea. He was evaluated by two physicians, both of whom concluded that he was experiencing aftershocks from his courtroom experience. During one examination, his blood pressure was elevated, but this finding was ignored.
>
> The symptoms persisted, and finally—quite reluctantly—the man agreed to his family's request that he see a third physician. By this time, he had lost 25 pounds and had become virtually homebound. He was tremulous, apprehensive, and thin with clammy palms. A full-scale medical workup for persistent diarrhea was conducted. Radiographic studies of the abdomen and kidneys showed an abnormal mass over the right kidney. At surgery an adrenal tumor, a pheochromocytoma, was removed.
>
> Ten months later, the man had regained his normal weight. He had become outgoing again and his general well-being was vastly improved. (Doust, 1958)

Pheochromocytoma is a rare tumor of the portion of the adrenal gland that secretes the body's natural stimulants. The tumor produces excessive amounts of catecholamines, sometimes episodically but in other instances continuously, as was true in the previous case; the individual, consequently, feels a sense of anxiety. This troubling mood is often accompanied by an elevated pulse rate, hypertension, excessive perspiration, severe headache, and diarrhea. Because this tumor is not usually malignant, surgical removal is curative.

Coffee, cola, and tea are heavily consumed by the American public. These popular drinks contain caffeine which is an effective stimulant. Individual sensitivity to caffeine is highly variable, but when a person has exceeded his individual threshold, nervousness, irritability, agitation, tremulousness, headaches, and palpitations are apt to appear.

Caffeine is not restricted to popular drinks. It is also an ingredient in chocolate and numerous over-the-counter preparations. Unknowingly, persons can get hooked on caffeine. When consumption is stopped or reduced (as may happen on weekends for many persons who consume excessive coffee during the work week), apathy and depression develops (often with headache) and drives the person to resume consuming caffeine.

An ambitious, hard-driving lieutenant colonel in the Army was referred from a military medical clinic to an outpatient psychiatric service for the evaluation of chronic anxiety.

As a daily occurrence for almost 2 years, the man had experienced symptoms of dizziness, tremulousness, apprehension, and difficulty sleeping. His repeated scores on the Hamilton Anxiety Scale were significantly elevated. Complete medical workups had been reported as normal on three occasions.

Treatment with Librium for 10 months followed by a 4-month trial on Valium had proved fruitless. The man's comment regarding these medications was that he disliked them because they "impaired his occupational precision."

On close questioning it was discovered that this 37-year-old lieutenant colonel regularly consumed 8–14 cups of coffee daily. He stated: "My coffee pot is a permanent fixture on my desk." In addition, prior to going to bed he habitually drank hot cocoa as a way of relaxing. His soft drink preference was cola. He drank 3–4 bottles a day. His total daily caffeine intake was roughly 1200 mg.

When confronted with the fact that he was suffering from caffeine toxicity (caffeinism), the lieutenant colonel at first expressed total disbelief and was unwilling to alter his caffeine intake even on a trial basis. Shortly thereafter, he reluctantly reconsidered. Within 4 weeks of starting on a caffeine-restricted diet, he showed a dramatic improvement in his tremulousness, insomnia, and other troublesome physical symptoms. To prove the causal relationship, his doctor reintroduced caffeine which led to a prompt return of symptoms.

Several months later—having returned to a caffeine-restricted diet—the man scored considerably lower on the Hamilton Anxiety Scale. Subjectively, he was free of anxiety and had shown no decline in his job performance. (Greden, 1974)

Cases of anxiety involving persons who regularly consume the daily equivalent of 800 mg of caffeine or more should be evaluated carefully for the possibility of caffeinism. Table 3.1 lists the caffeine content of some common substances.

The equating of "psychological" symptoms with psychological causation is an unsound clinical practice. Paranoia, depression, mania, and anxiety as well as a host of other mental manifestations can result from either psychological problems or organic disorders. As symptoms, they are indistinguishable. It is the overall context in which they appear—clinical history, related symptoms, risk factors—that will often indicate an organic cause.

TABLE 3.1 Caffeine Chart

Substance	Caffeine content in milligrams
Coffee	
Brewed	100–150/cup
Instant	85–100/cup
Tea	60–75/cup
Cola	40–60/cup
OTC Drugs	Variable, but often 100 mg/tab

GETTING SEDUCED BY THE STORY

Various versions of this clinical trap stem from the same basic mistake: accepting the "obvious" story without considering the rest of the facts.

Sometimes a previously established diagnosis sets the stage for this clinical mistake. The typical example goes like this: A person presents with characteristic symptoms. A review of the person's history shows previous episodes. Conclusion: the person is having the same psychological problem. Open and shut case! Right? Wrong!

The clinician should never forget that people frequently have more than one problem at a time. As clinicians we are prone to look for a single, all-encompassing explanation, but this is not always the case. Psychological and organic problems sometimes exist side by side. There is nothing to prevent a person with a serious problem in living from being physically ill at the same time. Failure to entertain this possibility is the source of serious clinical mistakes. You will recall that in a study of psychiatric outpatients, researchers discovered that 46% suffered from previously undiagnosed medical illnesses (Hall, Popkin, Devaul, Faillace, & Stickney, 1978).

> A 38-year-old woman with a well-documented history of manic-depressive disorder complained of fatigue, weight gain, and a strange sensitivity to cold weather, something she had not experienced before. She complained that upon washing her hair in the mornings, her drain became clogged with large amounts of hair.
>
> The woman had been maintained on lithium carbonate for three years with splendid results in controlling her mood swings. It was her psychiatrist's impression that now she was showing early, breakthrough signs of a depressive episode. (Jefferson, 1979)

This turned out to be a false assumption. Fatigue, weight gain, sensitivity to cold, and thinning of hair are characteristic manifestations of a deficient thyroid gland (hypothyroidism). In this case, the hypothyroidism was the result of prolonged use of lithium. Once she was started on replacement thyroid hormone, the patient's troublesome symptoms disappeared, despite her continuing on her medication.

Sometimes we become so preoccupied with getting "the story" we fail to make critical observations of a person's outward physical appearance. Such observations may provide important clues to an unexpected organic disease. When found in combination with physical disease, psychological symptoms should always be assessed for possible organic causes. Sometimes physical symptoms will have no connection, but this cannot be assumed. The clinician's best defense against neglecting physical findings is to develop a systematic approach to looking for them.

Table 3.2 lists some of the more readily observable physical findings that, although not invariably associated with organic disease, should be interpreted as strongly indicative. The listing is not comprehensive, but it does give the clinician a practical starting point.

Reading through the list, you may be slightly overwhelmed at the number of observations that should be made. Once a routine is established, however, these observations can be made unobtrusively in a relatively short time. Listening carefully to what a patient says is not incompatible with physical assessment. Failure to detect organic mental disorders frequently stems from overlooking the obvious.

A special instance of getting seduced by the story occurs around the issue of medical clearance. The clinician should never ignore findings suggestive of an organic problem simply because the person has been examined previously by a physician and "medically cleared." When a person is evaluated, the examination will only reveal what is detectable *at that particular time.* Physical diseases frequently have periods during which clinical detection is virtually impossible. Even highly sensitive laboratory tests will fail to detect disease at an early stage. After a person has been medically examined and referred for therapy, enough time may have elapsed for the problem to become manifest. Trust your observational skills. If signs of physical disease are present, do not let a previous medical clearance prevent you from calling for a reevaluation.

Medical clearance should always be viewed as *tentative,* subject to new evidence.

Unfortunately, sometimes medical evaluations are performed by incompetent physicians. The medical profession is not dissimilar to other professions. There are competent and incompetent practitioners, and on the surface, at least, it may be difficult to distinguish them. Failure to diagnose a

TABLE 3.2 Outward Manifestations of Physical Disease

Symptoms	Disease or condition
Overall appearance	
Dishevelment, gross errors in clothes selection	Various causes of brain syndrome
Movement	
Tremors, jerkiness, twitching, flinging motions, rigidity	Parkinson's disease, Huntington's chorea, tardive dyskinesia, Tourette's Syndrome
Disturbances in gait	Intoxications, cerebellar disease, normal pressure hydrocephalus
Head	
Cuts, abrasions, lumps, dried blood about the ear	Head trauma
Face	
Asymmetries in movement	Stroke
Eyes	
Bulging	Hyperthyroidism; tumors of the orbit behind the ear
Drooping eyelids	Myasthenia gravis (made famous by Aristotle Onassis); selective nerve dysfunction
Difference in pupil size	Brain masses (i.e., brain tumor, hematoma, abcess)
Widely dilated	Numerous drugs, particularly hallucinogens, stimulants, and anticholinergics
Markedly constricted	Opiate drugs (heroin, morphine)
Nonalignment of eyes (not parallel)	Dysfunction in cranial nerves innervating the eye muscles
Neck	
Protruding lumps	Thyroid enlargement, aneurysm of major arteries of the neck, cancerous growths
Skin	
Color changes, pallor "yellowing" (jaundice)	Anemia, shock diseases of the liver and gallbladder, cancer of the pancreas, acute anemia
Blue lips	Inadequate oxygenation as seen in certain heart and lung diseases
"Butterfly" rash (nose and face area)	Autoimmune diseases

TABLE 3.2 *(Continued)*

Symptoms	Disease or condition
Black and blue marks	Trauma, blood clotting deficiencies
Lines of discoloration	Needle tracks from drug mainlining
Thickening	Hypothyroidism
Excessive perspiration	Certain drugs, hypoglycemia and hypermetabolic conditions such as hyperthyroidism
Hair	
Extremely coarse and dry	Hypothyroidism
Extremely fine and silky	Hyperthyroidism

physical disease may not be a function of the invisibility of the disease, but rather the result of an inadequate examination. In addition, even the most capable of physicians have bad days. The signs of organic disease may simply be missed, an honest error which, nevertheless, can be tragic if it is neglected because "the doctor said there was nothing wrong."

Finally, the shifting nature of organic disease—especially organic brain syndromes—creates the distinct possibility of symptoms being absent at the time of examination. Later, perhaps even after a very brief period, the symptoms return and become readily observable.

> A young teacher, 26 years old, complained of spells of confusion and anxiety. At the initial medical evaluation, it was discovered that the woman was in the midst of a divorce and had been disowned by her family for living with a man they felt was "beneath" her. The woman was referred for supportive therapy.
>
> After her condition failed to improve, a more thorough medical evaluation showed that the patient had difficulty doing simple calculations. She also had trouble expressing herself, and her vision was impaired. Further studies led to a diagnosis of stroke, from which the woman fully recovered. (Weissberg, 1979)

What appeared to be a reaction to a stressful life was in fact an organic disorder stemming from circulatory blockage to the brain. The correct diagnosis was made after the woman had erroneously been medically cleared.

The moral for the clinician is this: Look and trust what you see. Even if the client has been previously cleared medically, a repeat evaluation may be indicated.

EQUATING PSYCHOSIS WITH SCHIZOPHRENIA (OR FUNCTIONAL PSYCHOSIS)

Equating psychotic behavior with schizophrenia is a serious and all too common clinical mistake. Although schizophrenia is the best known form of psychosis, it is by no means the only form. Psychosis most frequently arises from organic disorders. *In the absence of a well-established history of schizophrenia or bipolar disorder, any case of psychotic behavior should be considered organic until proven otherwise.*

If any of the core manifestations of brain syndrome (discussed in Chapter 4) are present, the diagnosis of schizophrenia should be questioned. This is not to say that such symptoms are never part of the clinical picture of schizophrenia. Sometimes confusion, disorientation, and recent memory deficits occur with schizophrenia, but when this is the case it is usually temporary, reflecting the patient's inattentiveness and distractibility. If symptoms of brain syndrome persists, further evaluation is essential to rule out a causative organic condition.

There is another point to keep in mind. Although brain syndrome is frequently encountered in cases of organic psychosis, exceptions are numerous. Its absence should not be construed as unquestionable proof of schizophrenia or other functional psychosis.

> A 31-year-old, fifth-year medical student claimed that he could read other people's minds and could hear his own internal thoughts spoken aloud. He thought that he was the son of a professor of psychiatry whom he believed to be disguised as the Duke of Gloucester. He suffered from an embarrassing compulsion to look at men "below the waist" and feared people thought he was homosexual.
>
> The young man's symptoms had emerged over a four-month period and intensified shortly after his wife gave birth to a second child. He began to feel that he was being hypnotized against his will.
>
> During a mental status examination, the patient saw the face of a dead relative smiling at him. He was, however, fully oriented. There was no previous history of mental disorder. (Bell, 1965)

This patient could easily have been misdiagnosed as schizophrenic, but further investigation documented an extensive use of amphetamines. He was suffering from an organic psychosis (without symptoms of brain syndrome) caused by chronic stimulant abuse.

In summary, psychosis with brain syndrome should be considered organic until disproven. Psychosis without brain syndrome may also be organic and should not be labeled schizophrenia without a complete evaluation.

There are several additional points of differentiation between functional psychosis and organic psychosis, although none are totally reliable. Persons experiencing schizophrenic symptoms for the first time usually are in their late teens or early twenties. Psychosis appearing for the first time in a person over the age of thirty is almost assuredly *not* schizophrenia. Serious errors in clinical assessment arise out of failure to consider this basic guideline.

Hallucinations are commonly encountered in psychosis. These distorted sensory experiences can involve any of the primary senses: sight, sound, touch, smell, or taste. Visual hallucinations are particularly characteristic of organic psychoses; less so of schizophrenia and other functional psychoses. But any form of hallucination can be seen in organic mental disorder. In fact, hallucinations (except for the hearing of voices) contrary to popular belief, are usually organic in origin.

Another differentiating feature is adaptive style (Golden et al., 1967). In functional psychosis, the familiar tends to be perceived as unfamiliar. This might, for example, result in the person's perceiving an old and trusted friend as a spy or an agent of the FBI. Organic psychosis is characterized by the opposite tendency: mistaking the unfamiliar for the familiar. This might lead to mistaking a total stranger for a friend or relative.

It is as though a sense of control is maintained in functional psychosis by attributing special—even bizarre—meaning to common things; whereas in organic psychosis, control is retained by translating (erroneously) the unknown or unrecognized into the familiar. Illusions—distorted perceptions— are instances of making the unfamiliar, familiar. They are characteristic of organic psychosis and rarely occur in schizophrenia.

The ability to get outside of oneself and to view one's experience objectively is completely disrupted in psychosis, but the waxing and waning of consciousness that characterizes organic psychosis produces momentary returns of self-awareness (Taylor, Maurer, & Tinklenberg, 1970). The person may express great concern over his mental condition: "Something terrible is wrong with me. This is not like me." Rarely is this seen in functional psychosis.

Certain forms of behavior have come to be equated with schizophrenia erroneously. Take catatonia, for example. Muscle rigidity with bizarre posturing, negativism, and mutism, in fact, is seen in numerous medical conditions having nothing to do with schizophrenia (Galenberg, 1976). A partial listing of organic problems causing catatonia includes:

viral encephalitis (limbic system)

brain tumors (frontal lobe and third ventricle)

petit mal epilepsy

head injuries

Wernicke's encephalopathy

syphilitic brain disease

narcolepsy

diabetic ketoacidosis

hypercalcemia

pellagra

acute intermittent porphyria

drug intoxications

paraneoplastic encephalopathy

Catatonia results from certain psychiatric medications, particularly the higher potency narcoleptic drugs. This finding is not particularly surprising. Catatonic-like rigidity in laboratory animals is one of the major screening criteria used by pharmaceutical manufacturers to identify substances with neuroleptic potential.

The clinical picture is dramatically eye-catching. The person appears frozen in space, reminiscent of the ray-gun effect portrayed in science fiction movies. A fixed posture may be maintained for hours. Characteristically, the person is mute. Extreme muscle tension is present, particularly about the face and in the muscles of the arms and legs. Heart rate and blood pressure are elevated and may be accompanied by excessive perspiration and fever. During periods when the person is not assuming a rigid posture, his walking may be stiff or labored. If the person speaks at all, the words may be sluggish and barely audible. Peculiar grimacing occurs intermittently. Despite the withdrawn appearance of catatonia, an underlying sense of hostility and obstinacy ("negativism") is present and may break through in violent outbursts, followed by a resumption of frozen posture.

The presence of catatonic behavior signals a serious disruption, but it says nothing per se about the cause. It does not automatically imply schizophrenia, as illustrated in the following case.

A graduate chemistry student awakened complaining of ringing in his ears. Within 30 minutes, after an episode of nausea and vomiting, he became confused. Alarmed, his wife rushed him to a hospital emergency room.

By the time he was examined, he had become belligerent, uncooperative, and even violent. Gradually, the clinical picture changed to one of incoherence and fearfulness. Upon admission, he was described as mute and drowsy. His heart rate was slightly elevated.

Over the next few hours the patient was observed by three staff psychiatrists who happened to be making medical rounds. They described a fluctuating clinical picture, cycling approximately every 20 minutes, from extreme, agitated excitement to stuporous catatonia with mutism. A provisional diagnosis was made of schizophrenia reaction, catatonic type.

The patient received a modest dose of a neuroleptic drug and promptly fell asleep. Twelve hours later he awakened fully coherent, cooperative, and speaking normally.

He reported being in excellent health until 3 days prior to admission, when he began working with a chemical—difluoronitroacetyl fluoride—in a poorly ventilated chemistry laboratory. After first experiencing numbness in his fingers, he awakened on the day of admission with the symptoms which led to his hospitalization.

The patient was discharged with a revised diagnosis of acute organic brain syndrome, secondary to organic fluoride poisoning. At a follow-up visit one year later, no residual symptoms or further episodes of catatonic behavior were reported. (Schwab & Barrow, 1964)

With respect to delusional thinking, the clinician should not assume that organic delusions will be devoid of specific, "dynamic" content. Organic delusions can be highly specific (Cummings, 1988). Delusional themes found in organic psychoses include the following:

- A loved one has been replaced by a clone-like imposter (Capgras syndrome)
- Unseen and unwelcome guests are living in the person's house (phantom boarder syndrome)
- The person is episodically transformed into a wolf (Lycanthropy or werewolfism)
- A lover is unfaithful (Othello syndrome)
- The person is infested with bugs (parasitosis)
- A mysterious persecutor constantly changes forms (Fregoli syndrome)
- The person is secretly loved by a celebrity (de Clarambault syndrome or erotomania).

A final point to consider relates to Schneiderian first-rank symptoms. Although often discussed relative to schizophrenia, these unusual manifestations are *not* unique to functional psychosis. Hearing one's thoughts broadcast out loud, feeling that one's thoughts are being involuntarily inserted (or extracted), or sensing one's feelings or actions emanating from an outside force—such delusions centering around the idea of alien influence occur in organic psychosis as well as in schizophrenia. They have no clinical differentiating value with respect to causal determination.

RELYING (UNNECESSARILY) ON LIMITED INFORMATION

The assessment of psychiatric problems is sometimes based on information from one source: the person coming for help. In such cases clinicians must proceed as best they can in arriving at some understanding of the problem. Frequently, however, the absence of other information or another perspective misleads the clinician. When information can be supplemented (particularly in cases where the person is intoxicated, confused, incoherent, or perhaps even comatose), it is essential to utilize additional resources. The true nature of a puzzling case may become readily apparent when supplementary information is obtained from other persons or clinical records.

Information from additional sources protects the clinician from several potential errors. It often clarifies aspects of the case that simply are not known to the patient; or even if known (because of the person's condition), cannot be recalled or accurately reported. It also protects the clinician against the patient's blind spots. The patient who does not want to face his problem may unconsciously suppress the facts, or attempt to minimize his deficits. Getting another perspective from someone who knows the person often makes obvious what may have been missed during a brief interview.

Even if a clinician is skilled at recognizing deception in the interview situation, the shifting presentation of brain syndrome (where symptoms appear and then disappear temporarily) is enough to give anyone pause. It is quite possible for an interview to take place when a patient, momentarily, has it all together. If a relative or friend, however, reports that the person has been getting lost over the past month, the clinician's perception of the problem will likely change.

Information obtained from other sources is particularly critical in cases of alcohol and drug abuse. Substance abusers are notorious for minimizing their problems. Their families may be falling apart, their jobs slipping away, their physical health failing; still they may deny having a problem with drinking or drugs.

Because substance abusers are at high risk for a variety of organic (as well as psychological) problems, information from another perspective is often invaluable. In the following case, supplementary information proved life-saving.

> A 23-year-old man with a history of severe alcoholism was seen in an emergency room for drunkenness. He appeared groggy; his speech was slurred. Intermittently, he fell asleep.
>
> The man had been accompanied by his wife, who assumed that he was probably "drinking again." On closer questioning, however, she said that her

husband's alcohol consumption over the past 24 hours actually had been quite minimal. She also recalled that on the preceding day her husband (while intoxicated) had fallen down the stairs in their home, after which he was unconscious for several minutes.

This additional history from the wife prompted further neurological testing that led to a diagnosis of subdural hematoma. The clot was evacuated by surgery, and the patient fully recovered. (Cadoret & King, 1974)

We have considered four clinical traps—mistaking symptoms for their causes, getting seduced by the story, equating psychosis with schizophrenia, and relying on limited information. Avoiding these traps is essential to the clinical recognition of psychological masquerade.

REFERENCES

Bell, D. S. (1965). Comparison of amphetamine psychosis and schizophrenia. *British Journal of Psychiatry, III*, 701–707.

Cadoret, R., & King, L. (1974). *Psychiatry and primary care.* St. Louis: C. V. Mosby.

Cummings, J. L. (1988). Organic psychosis. *Psychosomatics, 29*, 16–26.

Cummings, J., & Mendez, M. (1984). Secondary mania with focal cerebrovascular lesions. *American Journal of Psychiatry, 141*, 1084–1087.

Daley, R., Kane, F., & Ewing, J. (1967). Psychosis associated with the use of sequential oral contraceptive. *Lancet ii*, 444–445.

Doust, B. (1958). Anxiety as a manifestation of pheochromocytoma. *Archives of Internal Medicine, 102*, 811–815.

Erikson, E. (1963). *Childhood and society.* New York: Norton.

Galenberg, A. J. (1976). The catatonic syndrome. *Lancet, i*, 1339–1341.

Golden, J., Liston, E., Rimer, D., Rose, A., Sogher, D., & Solomon, D., (1967). Toxic and functional psychoses. *Annals of Internal Medicine, 66*, 989–1007.

Greden, J. (1974). Anxiety or caffeinism: a diagnostic dilemma. *American Journal of Psychiatry, 131*, 1089–1092.

Hall, R., Popkin, M., Devaul, R., Faillace, L, & Stickney, S. (1978). Physical illness presenting as psychiatric disease. *Archives of General Psychiatry, 35*, 1315–1320.

Illowsky, B., & Kirch, D. (1988). Polydipsia and hyponatremia in psychiatric patients. *American Journal of Psychiatry, 145*, 675–683.

Jefferson, J. (1979). Lithium carbonate-induced hypothyroidism, its many faces. *JAMA, 242*, 271–272.

Lewis, D., Comite, F., Mallouh, C., Zadunaisky, L., Hutchinson-Williams, K., Cherksey, B., & Yeager, C. (1987) Bipolar mood disorder and endometriosis: preliminary findings. *American Journal of Psychiatry, 144*, 1588–1591.

Rosenbaum, J., Tothman, J., & Murray, G. (1979). Psychosis and water intoxication. *Journal of Clinical Psychiatry, 40*, 287–291.

Rosenthal, N. E., Sack, D. A., Gillin J. C., Lewy, A., Goodwin, F., Davenport, Y., Mueller, P., Newsome, D., & Wehr, T. (1984). Seasonal affective disorder: a description of the syndrome and preliminary findings with light therapy. *Archives of General Psychiatry, 41*, 72–80.

Ryback, R., & Schwab, R. (1971). Manic response to levodopa therapy, report of a case. *New England Journal of Medicine, 285*, 788–789.

Schwab, J., & Barrow, M. (1964). A reaction to organic fluorides simulating classical catatonia. *American Journal of Psychiatry, 120*, 1196–1197.

Shulman, R. (1977). Psychogenic illness with physical manifestations and the other side of the coin. *Lancet, i*, 524–526.

Talbott, J., & Teague, J. (1969). Marijuana psychosis. *JAMA, 210*, 299–302.

Taylor, R., Maurer, J., & Tinklenberg, J. (1970). Management of "bad trips" in an evolving drug scene. *JAMA, 213*, 422–425.

Torrey, E. F. (1972). *The mind game: witchdoctors and psychiatrists.* New York: Emerson.

Vieweg, W., David, J., Rowe, W., Wampler, G., Burns, W., & Spradlin, W. (1985). Death from self-induced water intoxication among patients with schizophrenic disorders. *Journal Nervous Mental Disease, 173*, 161–165.

Weissberg, M. (1979). Emergency room medical clearance: an educational problem. *American Journal of Psychiatry, 136*, 787–790.

Chapter 4

A First Step: Recognition of Brain Syndrome

The harbingers are come. See, see their mark . . .   —George Herbert

From the outset, I need to emphasize that brain syndrome is *not* a specific disease; rather, it is the clinical expression of widespread brain failure associated with various conditions including drug toxicity, tumors, infections, degenerative brain diseases, hypertension, endocrine disorders, and nutritional deficiencies.

The recognition of brain syndrome is essential to the detection of psychologial masquerade because brain syndrome is highly correlated with organic disorders. Once identified, brain syndrome must be medically evaluated to determine the precise cause. It is the underlying, causative disease that must be treated, not the symptomatic manifestations. Although psychological reactions (particularly depression in the elderly) can sometimes assume the characteristics of brain syndrome, this is the exception. In fact, brain syndrome is so likely a reflection of organic disease that, in its presence, organicity must be assumed until proven otherwise.

Brain syndrome is a common clinical presentation. In this country one out of five patients admitted to a mental hospital has these symptoms. Studies of elderly persons *living in the community* have demonstrated a prevalence of 10–20%. In mental hospitals 50% of elderly persons have brain syndrome (Selzer & Sherwin, 1978).

It is essential to keep in mind that the causes of brain syndrome are sometimes reversible. Unfortunately, failure to recognize brain syndrome is a frequent clinical error. In one study of moderate-to-severe brain syndrome, the family physician failed to identify the problem in more than 80% of the cases (Williamson et al., 1964).

51

A word of caution. The reader should not fall into the trap of looking for brain syndrome only among the aged. The rise of drug and alcohol use in a younger population has created a substantial basis for brain syndrome. Also, increasingly, AIDS is a cause of brain syndrome among young adults.

A confusing terminology has developed. Dementia, delirium, acute and chronic organic brain syndrome, toxic psychosis, senility, presenility—all these terms have been used to refer to brain syndrome. Instead of clarifying the concept, however, this string of terms has created semantic chaos. For our purposes we will use the following definition. *Brain syndrome is a clinical presentation characterized by one or more of four cognitive deficits, occurring in varying combinations and resulting from a variety of causes.* If the reader starts with this broad working definition, the material that follows will fill in critical details. This characterization of brain syndrome integrates the *Diagnostic and Statistical Manual of Mental Disorders*, Third Edition, revised (American Psychiatric Association, 1987) categories of Organic Mental Disorders, providing—one hopes—a more practical scheme for organizing clinical observations.

The clinical picture of brain syndrome is greatly influenced by the rate of onset. If the compromise in brain functioning occurs rapidly, the outward manifestations are typically dramatic and severely disruptive. On the other hand, if the causative condition is slow in developing, a much more subtle clinical picture emerges, one which may remain hidden for some time. Although differing in clinical presentation, all variations of brain syndrome are characterized by deficits in one or more of four cognitive functions: *orientation, recent memory, reasoning, and sensory discrimination.*

Scattered throughout this chapter, the reader will find selections from a moving account of a 49-year-old academic researcher who developed brain syndrome secondary to Parkinson's disease, at a time when there was no effective treatment. It is taken from an article written by the man's son entitled "Death of a Mind: A Study in Disintegration."

> I first remember my father as a well-built, active man with a wide range of interests. His work required both intellectual and practical ability, and those who could judge his achievement spoke highly of it. I was more impressed at the time by the happy enthusiasm with which he would turn from weightier matters to entertain his small daughter . . . Over the period that we worked together, sometime in the early 1930s, I became gradually aware that the fine edge of his intellect was becoming dulled. He was less clear in discussion and less quick to make a jump from a new piece of evidence to its possible significance . . . He tended also to become portentous and solemn about his subject, as though one small corner of knowledge nearly filled his world, and the wider horizons were narrowing in. (Anonymous author, 1950)

COGNITIVE DEFICITS

In this book I distinguish schizophrenia and bipolar disorder from organic mental disorders. This is done despite the fact that considerable evidence has accumulated pointing the way to a biogenetic explanation for these conditions. With respect to clinical assessment, however, these so called "functional" psychoses differ from organic mental disorders. Many of the clues highly suggestive of organicity—such as brain syndrome—are absent. It is essential that specific organic mental disorders not be mistakenly labeled schizophrenia or manic-depressive psychosis, as this will deter the search for the true causative conditions. This differentiation is crucial to the recognition of psychological masquerade.

We need to begin our discussion of brain syndrome by taking up the problem of *inattention*. The ability to attend to the matter at hand is a basic prerequisite for normal behavior. There are many organic conditions *and* psychological states that severely compromise this function, making it impossible to maintain one's attention for any sustained period. The result is a frequent shifting from one concern or stimulus to another. Thinking, listening, performing—none of these is effective without the ability to attend; otherwise, moment to moment, one distraction after another makes it impossible to concentrate. Clinically, the inattentive person's face may dramatically communicate difficulty focusing for even the briefest period. His eyes may dart about, and his facial expression abruptly change. There may be extreme restlessness. The person may be continuously shifting, talking about one thing, then another and another and another.

When a person is having more subtle difficulty attending, a brief test known as "digit span retention" can be utilized to assess this problem more objectively. The person is asked to listen to a five-digit number and to repeat it immediately. Five random digits, such as 9-4-1-6-3, are presented, allowing approximately one second between numbers. Most adults perform this test without errror; if not, the test should be repeated, using a different set of digits. Failure on two attempts is strong evidence of inattention.

When an individual is having trouble attending, clinical assessment for brain syndrome becomes highly problematic because the ability to attend is an essential requisite to orientation, recent memory, basic reasoning, and sensory discrimination. The presence of severe inattention makes appraisal of the four cognitive deficits of brain syndrome difficult, if not impossible. False positives are to be expected. Reevaluation at a time when the person is more attentive (if this occurs) is indicated.

Disorientation

Orientation is the positioning of oneself with respect to time, space, and person. Disorientation frequently occurs as an early sign of brain syndrome. Sometimes without any significant disturbance in orientation a person may not know the *exact* date; but, there should be no difficulty identifying the correct month, year, and whether it is night or day. The inability to do so is evidence that a person is truly disoriented.

Disorientation to place is simply not knowing where you are. Normally, specifying where one is at any given moment should present no problem to a person, whether it is home, workplace, hospital, clinic, or jail. Brain syndrome often disrupts this basic orientation. Disorientation to place can best be evaluated in the actions of the person. Is there a history of the person's wandering about, unable to find the way home? Or, if the person is being observed as a patient, does he lose his way on the ward or go into the wrong room to sleep?

It is often said that, unlike disorientation to time and place, disorientation to person is rarely encountered in brain syndrome. If by this it is meant that there is no recognition of oneself, then this is true. If, however, disorientation to person is used to mean a failure to recognize people who should be familiar—relatives, friends, family physician, long-term therapist—then we are talking about a problem frequently seen in brain syndrome, although it is not as commonplace as time and place disorientation.

Orientation is a cornerstone of human experience. When a person becomes truly disoriented, brain disturbance is likely.

Recent Memory Impairment

Recent memory is the recall of an experience after a short time, say 5 to 10 minutes. Our memory system works by first registering (attending) an experience, then recording it (recent memory) and, finally, storing the information permanently for future retrieval (remote or long-term memory). As I discussed earlier, if a person cannot register (attend) the immediate experience, there is no possibility of its being recorded. Similarly, if an experience is registered but not recorded as a recent memory, it can never become permanently stored. In contrast, even when immediate and recent memory fail, old memories may be brought to mind, memories which were recorded years before. It is a disturbance in *recent memory* that is a hallmark of brain syndrome, whereas remote memory may or may not be compromised. Old memories may be recalled but new memories cannot be formed and, therefore, cannot be retained.

The easiest way to test recent memory is to list three unrelated items (key, stone, book) and inform the person that you will ask him to repeat them in a few minutes. Five minutes later the person should be able to recall the three items (not necessarily in the order presented). The examiner should not select words that can be connected through association (such as red and rose), as it is much less difficult to recall associated items.

Failure to recall three items after five minutes on two separate occasions indicates a recent memory defect. In addition to testing, the clinician should also be alert to a history of forgetfulness: missed appointments, repetition of stories or questions, leaving the stove on, or other oversights. This kind of "absentmindedness" suggests a disorder of recent memory.

> In 1935, after a period of absence, I looked forward with especial plea-sure to my homecoming, but when we met I knew with immediate cer-tainty that I had lost the companion of my earlier years. . . . To me it was as though a light had gone out, but no one else seemed to notice anything amiss. . . . We paused to consider a problem which had thwarted us, and I hit on a solution and outlined the idea. My father could not grasp the principle of it until I gave a demonstration. . . . I was profoundly shocked. . . . His ability was still well within normal limits; but I knew what it had been, and the difference was startling. . . . He tried to carry on with his work, but he did not make any headway and became more and more depressed about it. His character remained essentially the same except that he could no longer endure unorthodox views . . . if he chanced to overhear one of the eager iconoclastic arguments of youth, he became disturbed and petulant and it seemed as though his mental organization had become less secure even at its deeper levels. (Anonymous author, 1950)

Diminished Reasoning

A person's capacity to solve problems is diminished in brain syndrome. Friends or relatives may point out ridiculous mistakes made at home or on the job, mistakes seldom made prior to this time. A decline in basic reason-ing can make the solving of simple problems a difficult task. Making the correct change or keeping a golf score becomes difficult. Common sense judgment is lost. When asked what to do if accidentally locked out of the house or if in a car that has run out of gas, the person may become exas-perated and embarrassed, unable to come up with a reasonable answer.

Simple calculations are excellent devices for detecting deficits in prob-lem-solving.

- What remains if you subtract 7 from 22?
- How many eggs would you have if you had one-third of a dozen?
- If you wish to divide six books so that twice the number of books are on one shelf as on the other, how many books should you place on each shelf?

Brain syndrome tends to make these simple mathematical problems difficult to grasp and solve. But a word of caution. The clinician should keep in mind that memory and reasoning are *relative* skills. There is no single standard against which to measure them. Within the so-called "normal range," tremendous variation exists. For the particularly gifted, the task of recalling three items after 5 minutes or solving simple problems may create little difficulty *despite the presence of a mild brain syndrome.* Prior to the brain syndrome, however, the individual may have been able to recall ten items after 5 minutes as well as being able to solve highly complex problems. Thus, whereas failure on these simple screening questions is always suggestive of brain syndrome, success cannot be construed as conclusive evidence against brain syndrome. For this reason, the clinician should obtain information from relatives and friends about the patient's prior level of functioning as a context in which to interpret present performance. A history of deteriorating cognitive skills at home or work is highly significant regardless of the person's ability on screening tests.

Sensory Indiscrimination

During the course of day-to-day living, we are exposed to massive amounts of sensory input from the external world as well as from within. The brain must sort out this information, assigning priorities, and construing its meaning. Of all the sensory input we receive, only a relatively small amount can be actively considered; otherwise, we would become lost in a vast gulf of overstimulation. Our world of meaning would disintegrate into noise and confusion. A diminished capacity for sensory discrimination is found in brain syndrome. Selectivity fails; sensory overload threatens; and the misinterpretation of sensations results.

Within the emergence of brain syndrome, sensory indiscrimination typically takes the form of illusions. An illusion is the misidentification of an external stimulus: the mistaking of something for what it is not. For example, the individual may look at dimly lit curtains across the room gently moved by the wind and mistake them for a person. A street sound may be misinterpreted as the voice of a friend. This kind of perceptual distortion can involve any of the five senses—sight, sound, touch, taste and smell—

but, most often, illusions are visual or auditory. Illusions are *rarely* seen as psychological reactions; their presence indicates organicity.

Hallucination is a second form of sensory indiscrimination. In contrast to illusions, hallucinations are perceptual experiences that have *no* external referent. They are internal experiences projected onto the outside world. The person may hear a voice when no one is speaking, or see things—a face, spiders on the wall, snakes on the floor, a hooded demon—in the absence of any related external object. As with illusions, hallucinations occur in all sensory modes, but *visual* hallucinations are particularly common in brain syndrome. Visual hallucinations can be extremely terrifying to the individual; but, in other instances, the hallucinated experience may be a source of pleasure. One author has reported observing a person with brain syndrome who intently (and apparently with great pleasure) followed a 30-minute football game between two teams of miniature elephants! (Lishman, 1978.)

Although not as prevalent as visual hallucinations, other forms of hallucinations occur as part of brain syndrome. Tactile hallucinations (especially prevalent in cocaine withdrawal) may take the form of tiny creatures crawling over the skin. Olfactory hallucinations are often experienced in the initial phase of temporal lobe epilepsy. Typically, the person smells an awful odor, variously described as "rotten eggs," "burning rubber," or "old cheese."

Auditory hallucinations—a hallmark of schizophrenia—also sometimes occur in brain syndrome. When present, they are usually threatening or derogatory (Farber, 1959). Since auditory hallucinations are common in schizophrenia, they are a problematic indicator. The question arises, should the clinician consider any form of hallucination as indicative of organic brain disease?

As an approach to screening, the following rule can be used: *the presence of any hallucination—other than auditory—is presumptive evidence of an organic problem.* In the absence of other organic evidence, auditory hallucinations *alone* are not strongly indicative of an organic problem. The one major exception to this rule is seen in association with chronic alcoholism: a condition known as hallucinosis, characterized by the hearing of voices which are almost always threatening in nature.

> If my father glanced at a dark shape which was rather like a black cat, he did not instinctively look again to make sure what it was; he simply saw a cat. His mind fitted the sensory impression to the first rough approximation which suggested itself, and accepted it without further question, however unlikely it might be in the context. . . . My father discussed the problem with me in some detail, as he was naturally disturbed to find that he kept on seeing things which were not there. (Anonymous author, 1950)

BRAIN SYNDROME IN CONTEXT

We have considered four cognitive deficits found in varying combinations in brain syndrome. Now we need to fill in the picture further by considering the typical clinical presentations of brain syndrome.

There are two prominent versions of brain syndrome, and scattered along a continuum between them are a number of variations resembling one more than the other but usually incorporating aspects of each.

Rapid-Onset Brain Syndrome (ROBS)

> A request for an "emergency psychiatric consultation" was made a few days after the admission of a 35-year-old man to the hospital for treatment of pneumonia. The consultation request was accompanied by a brief clinical note stating that the patient had become "schizophrenic with hallucinations and delusions."
>
> When examined, the man appeared extremely agitated. He was restless, fidgeting with the bed coverings, and sometimes waving his arms inappropriately. Unable to attend to any task for more than a few moments, he was highly distractable and appeared frightened. Although he gave his name correctly, he seemed unaware that he was sick and in a hospital. When pressed on this matter, he said he thought he was in a bakery. Later, he said it was a bank.
>
> He gave the year as 1964, rather than 1971, and was unable to identify the month or day of the week. At times he responded as if he were seeing things. He thought there was an angel standing beside his bed, caring for him, but he wondered if it might not have been sent to harm rather than to protect him. (Sakles & Ballis, 1978)

This man was not suffering from schizophrenia. He was manifesting brain syndrome secondary to pneumonia. Likely this infection was preventing adequate oxygen from reaching his brain. The result: brain failure. As the pneumonia was brought under control with antibiotics, his mental symptoms cleared.

The most common causes of ROBS are drug and alcohol intoxications and the associated withdrawal states that develop. But many acute medical diseases, either through direct impairment of the brain or compromise of its support system, can also lead to ROBS.

Typically, ROBS manifests as a sudden, dramatic change in behavior. The individual will usually be disoriented to time and place and will be highly distractable, unable to focus on anything for more than a few seconds. If the person's attention can be captured long enough to test for recent memory, a severe deficit will be confirmed. The inability to concentrate makes simple problem-solving difficult, if not impossible. Overall, the person will project an appearance of confusion.

Misinterpretations of the surrounding environment, although often prominent, sometimes can be quite subtle. Hallucinatory experiences, particularly visual, may be obvious if a person turns his head to listen or suddenly shouts back to an empty room; but, in other instances, these hallucinatory experiences may be carefully masked by an individual in the grip of paranoia, afraid others will punish him or take advantage of him if his hallucinations are detected.

Restlessness is one of the earliest behavioral indicators of impending ROBS. In a classic study of "delirium," investigators found that some degree of restlessness was "invariably present." Restlessness can manifest in various ways, including being easily startled, pacing the floor, continually fumbling with one's clothes or bed covers, and repetitively searching for things (Wolff & Curran, 1935).

Tremulousness—a fine, quivering movement of the muscles—may be seen with ROBS (particularly in cases involving drugs or alcohol) and can accentuate the clinical picture of restlessness.

A tendency toward insomnia or a reversal of the sleep cycle so that what little sleep there is comes during the daylight hours is also commonly found.

The term *shifting level of consciousness* describes a striking characteristic of ROBS: one moment the person appears grossly confused, disoriented, and completely illogical; a few hours later, calm, rational, and in control. During this so-called lucid interval, the deficits associated with brain syndrome, if detectable at all, may be much less noticeable. But the improvement is only momentary, after which the manifestations of brain syndrome return in full force. One researcher described an encounter with a patient as he recovered in the hospital from back surgery (Lipowski, 1967). The man, a minister, greeted the physician researcher shouting that he had lost his genitals in a car accident. The next moment he was screaming that a dog was biting his penis. Suddenly, he shifted the conversation once again to a discussion of tropical flowers which he appeared to be hallucinating. After several more minutes of fragmented, one-way conversation, the man turned and said: "Am I sick? I seem to be hallucinating!" When told that this was true, he seemed relieved and remained quiet for a few minutes. Then he began to shout again: "Look, look, there's this dog again, biting me! Take the dog away!" This is an example of shifting level of consciousness, which to some degree characterizes most cases of ROBS.

ROBS can be influenced by environmental factors. It predictably worsens in the nighttime. Being left alone in a room, particularly one without windows, can also exacerbate ROBS, and individuals who have undergone surgery followed by convalescence in an intensive care unit develop ROBS with some degree of regularity, thought in part to result from relative sensory deprivation.

> *The suggestion that he should then go for a trip abroad put me in a difficult position. He felt convinced that it would do him good, and his medical advisors encouraged this belief. . . . We left England at the end of the year. Our destination was an isolated resort in mountainous country about fifteen miles from the nearest small town. . . . It was soon evident, however, that unfamiliar faces and a foreign language were putting too heavy a strain on his fading faculties. . . . Now, listening every day to a background of foreign conversation which, even when fit, he could not easily have followed, he was bewildered. . . . His mind accepted the nearest English equivalent to the sounds he heard, and the task of keeping in touch with reality against such odds became impossible. Hearing what he thought was English spoken, he addressed other hotel residents in his own language to be met by uncomprehending stares. He naturally came to feel that they were hostile to him, and he began gradually to make order out of his mental chaos by systematizing, in a delusional way, what he heard and saw. (Anonymous author, 1950)*

Two versions of ROBS have been described: one characterized by increased activity, the person appearing agitated, if not driven or frenzied; the other, by diminished activity, with an apathetic, withdrawn, or even drowsy appearance. This latter version of ROBS, because the person is not disruptive, is easily overlooked. Regardless of its type of presentation, ROBS should be considered a medical emergency requiring immediate evaluation.

Slow-Onset Brain Syndrome (SOBS)

This form of brain syndrome emerges insidiously. Contrasted to the sudden, rapidly developing clinical picture of ROBS, there is a slow, progressive deterioration in orientation and recent memory combined with a decline in common judgment and problem-solving skills.

Given the more gradual onset of SOBS, the person has time to adapt. Certain tasks may be avoided, particularly those that require recent memory and problem-solving. Social engagements are restricted. Eventually, however, the person loses his ability to hide the problem. Judgment becomes seriously compromised so that the person appears irresponsible and accident-prone. Difficulty grasping abstract or symbolic meaning becomes obvious. Jokes are no longer understood. Simple proverbs are perplexing. The person interprets them literally. Thus, the saying, "The grass is always greener on the other side," may lead the person with SOBS to comment on different kinds of grass or various shades of green rather than the idea that things we do not have often appear more attractive than things we do have. The same difficulty is observed when the person is asked to identify a characteristic shared by several different things. For example, given a list of five colors, the person may be unable to perceive that blue, red, pink, purple, and green are similar in that they are all colors. (The ability to abstract is also compromised in cases of ROBS, but this deficit is usually overshadowed by prominent behavioral changes. In schizophrenia, there is often a bizarre twist to the literal interpretation not typically found in SOBS.)

Of course the sketch I am presenting of SOBS is a composite; not all cases will include each clinical element.

Various organic conditions produce SOBS; some, such as Alzheimer's disease, permanently. Others, as we shall discuss later, are completely or partially reversible when appropriately treated. Although SOBS is more commonly seen among the elderly, it is by no means restricted to them.

Let me encourage the reader to pause for a moment and fantasize the experience of SOBS. What would be your personal response to an unexplainable failing memory, disorientation, and a breakdown in reasoning—all of which have been dependable aspects of your life heretofore? At first you might try to deny what was occurring, but with time, denial would be impossible in the face of accumulating evidence. Your self-confidence would diminish as the disturbing, if not terrifying, threat of losing control loomed. You would sense that something dreadful was wrong, but you would not understand precisely what it was. Even though you could no longer keep the truth from yourself, you might still try to hide it from others, hoping it would go away. You would stop putting yourself on display. Social engagements would be avoided, including perhaps the weekly card game you had enjoyed over the years.

Your checking account might turn up overdrawn—not once, but repeatedly. You lose track of important engagements. Even at home, conversation with family and friends becomes stressful. You are afraid of making a fool of yourself. Gradually, you say less and less, fading off into thinking about other things; but, when someone asks a question, you are forced to make up a response which provokes stares of bewilderment. As time goes on, more and more, you find yourself in situations that seem strange. You are not sure of what people are discussing or why they look at you and ask questions that make no sense. Things—familiar things—fleetingly appear different. Sometimes objects seem to come alive, but when you refocus, the animation is gone. You find it difficult to sleep. Restlessly, you toss and turn in bed, almost afraid of what might happen if you should fall asleep. Your vitality leaves you; you find no humor in experiences that others find hilarious. You feel hopelessly bewildered and frightened, unavoidably aware of your failing faculties.

> At the request of her family physician, a 78-year-old woman was seen in her home by a public health nurse. The woman had lived with her middle-aged daughter until recently, when the daughter required hospitalization for high blood pressure.
> The nurse observed that the house was messy and the woman unkempt. Throughout the conversation, the elderly woman kept insisting that her daughter had just stepped out briefly for a walk. She persisted in this story despite being told repeatedly that her daughter was in the hospital. When queried about the date, she missed it by two years.
> Three days later, the police escorted the woman to an emergency room, having found her wandering some distance from her home in her night clothes, "looking for my daughter."
> On examination she was unable to recall more than one of three objects after five minutes and failed to recognize the name of the current president. She insisted on referring to the physician as "Father," stating that she had not been to church enough lately. When asked the meaning of commonly used proverbs, she said they were "silly." In response to "a stitch in time saves nine," she replied that her eyes were "too weak to sew."
> She was suffering from senile dementia. (Horvath, 1979)

Dramatic changes in personality are seen with SOBS and, in some instances, may be the initial manifestation. These changes fall roughly into four clinical patterns. The person may show an exaggeration of certain personality traits. A previously compulsive person may become rigid and obstinate; a passive–dependent individual, demanding and infantile. A mildly nervous and anxious person may develop obsessive concerns over minor issues. In short, the person becomes a caricature of himself.

In some cases of SOBS this change in personality takes the form of excessive emotional displays, sometimes referred to as "lability of emotional expression." With the slightest provocation, the person may laugh hysterically or, as is more often the case, cry uncontrollably. These excessive emotional expressions are stereotypical in quality. Facial expressions tend to be exactly the same each time the person has one of these emotional outbursts. After a short time, the reaction subsides, only to return later at another inappropriate moment.

A second type of personality change involves restlessness, hyperactivity, loss of social discretion, and inappropriate bravado and euphoria which when restrained by others quickly evolves into angry agitation. This pattern can be mistaken for the manic phase of bipolar disorder.

The opposite personality change is also seen: apathy, social withdrawal, and depression. Many cases of SOBS are misinterpreted as instances of psychological depressive reactions.

A fourth type of personality change is characterized by growing suspiciousness that can become frank paranoia. Often, irrational jealousy will be a major element of the person's paranoid thinking.

When personality changes precede or overshadow the cognitive deficits of SOBS, the stage is set for psychological masquerade.

> He spent the days chasing non-existent spies in other people's bedrooms; while I chased after, explaining to the agitated guests and taking what steps I could to deal with the emergency . . . the situation forced me to restrain him. . . . In that moment of despair and disillusion the full force of his love for me was turned to bitter hatred. . . . When the crisis came we were alone in an upstairs gallery, and he turned on me with murder in his eyes. . . . For a moment the issue hung in the balance . . . but when my glance met his, he could not bring himself to do it. He relaxed at last with a gesture of sad acquiescence and let himself be quietly led away. (Anonymous author, 1950)

Table 4.1 provides a summary of the commonalities and differences of ROBS and SOBS including the issue of reversibility.

THE QUESTION OF REVERSIBILITY

Although SOBS can reflect irreversible brain deterioration, many cases result from conditions that, when correctly treated are partially or totally reversible.

A review of two sizable studies of "progressive intellectual deterioration" found that approximately one out of every four cases had "an underlying disease potentially reversible by medical or surgical therapy" (Freeman, 1967). A later study puts the figure even higher. Out of 222 cases of brain syndrome 35–40% were found through further medical evaluation to be treatable conditions (Wells, 1978). Persons with SOBS are all too frequently viewed as "crocks" or "senile" for whom nothing can be done. *SOBS should never be presumed irreversible until a thorough medical evaluation has been conducted*

A retired farm worker, aged 67, of sound physical and mental health, lost interest in activities that previously had given him considerable pleasure. His

TABLE 4.1 Brain Syndrome

ROBS	SOBS
Rapid, dramatic onset	Slow, subtle onset
Shifting level of consciousness	Downward progression
Usually reversible	Sometimes reversible

Core deficits
(One or more)

Disorientation
Recent memory impairment
Diminished reasoning
Sensory Indiscrimination

(Behavioral changes)	(Personality changes)
Examples	*Examples*
Acute drug intoxications	Hypothyroid psychosis
Encephalitis	Pernicious anemia
Drug withdrawal reactions	Alzheimer's disease

family found him distant and forgetful. One evening when he failed to return from his usual walk, a search of the surrounding area found him covered with mud, soaking wet, and extremely confused. It was assumed he had either deliberately or accidentally fallen into the nearby river. After a night's sleep, he seemed for the most part his usual self.

His family, however, remained concerned and finally insisted on a medical examination. This turned up "generalized rhonchi" in the man's chest. He was admitted to a hospital on the assumption that he had inhaled water when he had fallen into the river.

During his hospitalization, he appeared depressed. Although fully oriented, he answered questions slowly and with poor detail. His medical evaluation established a vitamin B_{12} deficiency (pernicious anemia). Treatment with B_{12} injections was immediately initiated. Within a few weeks, he showed great improvement. His mental alertness and spontaneity returned, and he experienced no further episodes of confusion. (Later, it was discovered that the man's brother also had suffered from pernicious anemia.) (Strachen & Henderson, 1965)

The Amnestic Syndrome (Amnesia)

The amnestic syndrome is a well-circumscribed form of brain syndrome. It is characterized by a profound alteration in orientation and recent memory

(Benson, 1978). While the person has no difficulty attending to the immediate situation and can readily solve simple problems, when he or she is tested for retention of new information, a striking defect is apparent. The ability to recall even one or two objects after 5 to 10 minutes is lost. The person is simply unable to hold onto recent experience; learning new information becomes impossible.

There is also a severe disorientation to time and place, reflecting the close tie between orientation and the assimilation of new information. Consequently, persons suffering from the amnestic syndrome are prone to lose their way; and, experientially, are continually "meeting" new people whom they have previously met and forgotten. Thus, this condition leaves the person quite capable of immediately recalling five digits and retrieving old memories out of the past, but, between old and immediate experience, a devastating memory void exists.

As a means of coping with a continual loss of new information, the person begins to confabulate; that is, to make up responses in order to fill the memory gaps. This results in the creation of fanciful, if not outrageous, tales that can be mistaken for psychotic delusions by the unsuspecting clinician.

The amnestic syndrome can arise from head trauma, stroke, oxygen deprivation, or a deficiency of thiamin (vitamin B_1) most often caused by chronic alcoholism. This alcohol-related amnesia is called Korsakoff's Syndrome, after the Russian physician who first described it in the late 1800s.

A 50-year-old man with a long-standing alcohol problem was hospitalized after several months of heavy drinking. The man had neglected his appearance and nutrition and had begun to talk to himself much of the time. When admitted to the hospital, he was noted to be "completely disoriented." He persisted in his contention that he had "been brought to the hospital after an injury to his leg at the shipyard," an event which, in actuality, had occurred 10 years earlier.

The day after he was transferred from one hospital building to another, the patient estimated that one week had passed since leaving the other building, and his memory for details of his initial hospital setting already had begun to fade. In contrast, the man's memory for past years remained relatively intact. He was able to recall the exact address of the boarding house where he had lived years before his hospitalization.

Despite his situation, the man would not admit that he had trouble remembering. Instead, during conversations he would make vague statements hoping they would appear consistent and logical. Sometimes, however, he would slip and make statements which were obviously untrue. When tested with three pictures, he could never recall the first two. Only memory of the third picture remained. At times when confronted with obvious contradictions, he would change his explanation. (Lidz, 1942)

In this chapter I have characterized brain syndrome as a variable clinical presentation involving one or more of four cognitive deficits: disorientation, recent memory impairment, diminished reasoning, and sensory indiscrimination. Recognizing these cognitive deficits is of considerable clinical import, since they are highly correlated with organic disease that in many instances may be correctable.

We have discussed two versions of brain syndrome—ROBS and SOBS—as well as the amnestic syndrome, an unusual variation of brain syndrome characterized by a striking deficit in recent memory and orientation. Although, to facilitate our review, ROBS and SOBS have been portrayed as separate clinical presentations, this clear demarcation is not always obvious in the day-to-day world of clinical practice. Persons with SOBS are prone to the superimposition of ROBS resulting from infections, medications, sensory deprivation, and nonspecific stress. In turn, ROBS may be the initial manifestation of a process that with time evolves into SOBS. The clinician should be familiar with these two clinical versions of brain syndrome and should realize that they often blend together.

Finally, we have reviewed various personality changes which may overshadow the presence of brain syndrome.

I once gave a two-hour lecture on brain syndrome and its importance in helping to differentiate organic from psychological disorders. At the conclusion, a student raised his hand and said, "I don't get it!" He went on to explain that all the "mental patients" he had seen acted confused and out of it. When I pushed him to give examples, he began to reel off instances of bizarre thinking: a man who thought he was king and a woman who felt she had gotten pregnant from watching television. His conclusion was that all psychiatric patients are "confused." "They don't know where they are or what's going on. They *all* have brain syndrome." Clearly, for this one student, I hadn't made my point. He still thought that "crazy" thinking was synonymous with brain syndrome; thus, before I conclude this chapter, let me make *the point* a final time.

Most people with psychological problems (the kind of problems for which people most often seek counseling or psychotherapy) are *not* disoriented. They are usually perfectly capable of solving simple problems and calculations and have intact recent memory. Other than auditory hallucinations (seen mainly in persons with schizophrenia), they are not suffering from gross sensory indiscrimination. Even in cases of schizophrenia or bipolar disorder, despite intensely painful emotions, severe stress or even psychotic thought, core cognitive functioning remains relatively intact as long as the person's attention can be elicited.

When a person exhibits brain syndrome, brain disease is the most likely explanation. The major exceptions are persons who are so inattentive that

TABLE 4.2 Brain Syndrome Deficits

Disorientation

Time: inability to identify the *month, year or general time of day (day or nighttime)*

Place: inability to identify one's *present location*

Person: inability to recognize *persons* who should be *quite familiar.*

Recent memory impairment

Failure to recall *three items* after *5 minutes* on *two* occasions.

Diminished reasoning

Inability to solve simple problems:

- What remains when you subtract 7 from 22?
- How many eggs would you have if you had one-third of a dozen?
- If you wish to divide six books so that twice the number of books are on one shelf as on the other, how many books should you place on each shelf?
- What would you do if you locked your keys in the car?

Sensory indiscrimination

The presence of *illusions* or *hallucinations* (other than isolated auditory hallucinations).

---

other cognitive functions are impossible to test adequately. Even schizophrenic persons when they are extremely bizarre in their thinking, if you can command their attention for a few minutes, will not manifest brain syndrome.

While some cases of brain disease will not cause brain syndrome, most instances of brain syndrome turn out to be the product of brain disease. The core brain syndrome deficits are summarized in Table 4.2

In the next chapter, we will consider additional clues to organic mental disorder that, along with recognition of brain syndrome, provide the clinician with a comprehensive approach to detecting psychological masquerade.

Once we got back to England, he was admitted to a mental hospital without delay. He had long since given up the struggle of trying to relate his ideas to reality, and had retired into a private world of unimpeded action. When last I saw him he had been put in charge of running the war after Dunkirk and was well pleased with the results. (Anonymous author, 1950)

REFERENCES

American Psychiatric Association (1987). *Diagnostic and statistical manual of mental disorders* (Third Edition Revised), Washington, D.C. American Psychiatric Association.

Anonymous. (1950). Death of a mind: a study in disintegration. *Lancet, i,* 1012–1015.

Benson, F. (1978). Amnesia. *Southern Medical Journal, 71,* 1221–1228.

Farber, I. (1959). Acute brain syndrome. *Diseases of the Nervous System, 20,* 296–299.

Freeman, F. (1967). Evaluation of patients with progressive intellectual deterioration. *Archives of Neurology, 33,* 658–659.

Horvath, T. (1979). Organic brain syndromes. In A. Freeman, R. Sack, & P. Berger (Eds.). *Psychiatry for the Primary Care Physician* (215–245). Baltimore: Williams and Wilkins.

Lidz, T. (1942). The amnestic syndrome. *Archives of Neurology and Psychiatry, 47,* 588–605.

Lipowski, Z.J. (1967), Delirium, clouding of consciousness and confusion. *Journal of Nervous and Mental Disease, 145,* 227–255.

Lishman, W. (1978). *Organic psychiatry.* London: Blackwell Scientific Publications.

Sakles, G.J. & Ballis, G. (1978). Acute brain syndromes. In G. Balis (Ed.). *Clinical Psychopathology* (pp. 65–86). Boston: Butterworth Publishers, Inc.

Selzer, B., & Sherwin, I. (1978). Organic brain syndromes: an empirical study and critical review. *American Journal of Psychiatry, 135,* 13–21.

Strachen, R.W., & Henderson, J.G. (1965). Psychiatric syndrome due to avitaminosis B_{12} with normal bone marrow. *Quarterly Journal of Medicine, 34,* 303–317.

Wells, C. (1978). Chronic brain disease: an overview. *American Journal of Psychiatry, 135,* 1–12.

Williamson, J., Stokoe, I.H., Gray, S., Fisher, M., Smith, A., McGhee, A., & Stephenson, E. (1964). Old people at home: Their unreported needs. *Lancet, i,* 1117–1120.

Wolff, H.G., & Curran, D. (1935). Nature of delirium and allied states. Archives of Neurology and Psychiatry, 33, 1175–1215.

Chapter 5

More Clues to Psychological Masquerade

Some circumstantial evidence is very strong, as when you find a trout in the milk.
—Henry David Thoreau

In this chapter we will consider two kinds of additional clues to psychological masquerade. *Alerting clues* sensitize the clinician to the need for a thorough search for organic mental disorder. The greater the number of these clues, the more intense the clinician's suspicion should be. *Presumptive clues* are even more compelling in their implication. Until proven otherwise (through medical evaluation), the presence of one or more presumptive clues (in association with psychological symptoms) should be interpreted as persuasive evidence of organicity. Brain syndrome, as we have already seen, is one presumptive clue to psychological masquerade, but there are several others that should be considered, for they may appear in the absence of brain syndrome.

ALERTING CLUES

We will consider five findings suggestive of organic mental disorder. None of these clues alone proves organicity, but their presence should sensitize the clinician to the possibility. Alerting clues serve as flashing red lights, and should heighten the search for organic mental disorder.

No History of Similar Symptoms

The initial occurrence of a psychological symptom should be carefully scrutinized. Generally, one of the best predictors of the future is the past; thus, if

69

a person has never heretofore reacted to the stresses and strains of living with psychiatric symptoms, the emergence of such symptoms should suggest the possibility of an alternative explanation.

> A 54-year-old woman with no previous history of mental illness suddenly experienced a "delirious" episode, lasting for almost 24 hours. Her confusion cleared, only to be replaced by changes in her mood and personality, manifest as depression and childlike dependency. After these changes worsened over a 10-month period, the woman was admitted to a hospital.
>
> She was diagnosed as suffering from depression and treated with ECT. During the course of her treatment, however, she developed obvious neurological deficits, including weakness in her left arm and leg. At surgery an inoperable brain tumor was discovered infiltrating the right frontal, temporal, and parietal areas of the brain. (Waggoner & Bagohi, 1954)

Particular attention should be given to the late manifestation of symptoms that ordinarily occur earlier in life. For example, "scchizophrenia" is sometimes loosely applied to any person who exhibits delusions or hallucinations. As previously mentioned, clinicians would be well advised to question this characterization of psychotic symptoms when they occur initially after the age of 30. Schizophrenia, in the vast majority of cases, manifests itself in the late teens and early twenties.

The emergence of new symptoms should also be suspect. A history of one kind of symptom should not automatically be assumed to relate to current symptoms. For example, previous episodes of bizarre behavior may have nothing to do with the subsequent emergence of paranoid confusion. The initial occurrence of any psychiatric symptom should always create some degree of suspicion of psychological masquerade.

No Readily Identifiable Cause

Mental and emotional symptoms arising in the context of a relatively trouble-free life should make the clinician uneasy. Even though the precise nature of the problem may remain unclear, in psychological reactions typically there are signs of stress in the person's life. Psychological changes that emerge without warning usually can be traced to a readily identifiable conflict or trauma. In contrast, organic mental disorders often appear abruptly "out of the blue," without explanation.

> The concerned friends of a 31-year-old computer sciences student brought the young man to an emergency room after his friends had observed strange behaviors in him over a 48-hour period. They related how he had abruptly

started to hear voices and had become quite withdrawn. He avoided conversations. When he did respond, he gave short, incomplete answers, seemingly unrelated to the discussion.

Further questioning of the friends revealed that a week before, the young man had dropped his studies and quit his job as a taxi driver. He had also complained of a headache for which he sought help from several physicians without relief.

The man was described as a loner, but with no history of mental disorder. No precipitating event for his current symptoms could be identified.

Although fully oriented, he had considerable difficulty complying with simple requests. He did not appear to understand the questions being asked and was thought by a psychiatrist to have "loosening of associations." His memory proved "difficult to test."

He was admitted to a psychiatric unit with a tentative diagnosis of "acute schizophreniform psychosis." (Carlson, 1977)

The abrupt onset of strange behavior (with no previous history of mental disorder) combined with poor cognitive functioning (as well as an unexplained headache) should have raised the suspicion of psychological masquerade. Within 24 hours the young man developed fever and a stiff neck. An emergency angiogram (a contrast study of the brain using dye that can be seen on x-ray) showed a large subdural hematoma. Reparative surgery was immediately performed with excellent results, leaving no residual symptoms. The hematoma had developed from a "leaking" artery, known as an "aneurysmal malformation," a somewhat rare congenital anatomical defect.

Although psychological symptoms in the absence of significant stress is suggestive of an organic mental disorder, *the reverse is not true.* The existence of problems in living cannot be taken as proof positive of a psychological reaction. As illustrated by numerous examples throughout this book, the most plausible psychological explanations are frequently identifiable in cases of organic mental disorder. *The fact that a sound psychological explanation can be advanced should not blind the clinician to evidence for an organic mental disorder.*

Age 55 or Older

Older persons are particularly prone to psychological masquerade. Organic mental disorders account for more than half the initial psychiatric admissions in persons age 55 or older.

Several factors contribute to this increased risk. First, the wide margins of safety within the support systems of the body decline with age; consequently, maintenance of an optimal physiological environment (on which brain functioning depends) is less dependable than in earlier years.

Second, the brain as we age becomes more sensitive to drugs and less adroit at adapting to troublesome side effects. Finally, the incidence of numerous diseases capable of psychological masquerade increases with age, as does the risk of accidental falls and head injury.

I do not mean to imply that psychological reactions are absent from older life. They do happen; but so do psychological masquerades, and they show a dramatic increase with age.

Coexistence of Chronic Disease

Persons suffering from chronic diseases commonly receive medications that can cause adverse effects resembling psychological symptoms. Also, long-standing chronic diseases frequently lead to physiological decline and failure. Of course, the degree of risk for organic mental disorder depends on the specific type of disease. Some chronic diseases create minimal risk while others often lead to organic mental disorders. Consider the following case.

> After the death of her husband, a 56-year-old woman (over the next 48 hours) became increasingly agitated. When she insisted that her brother was her dead husband returned to life, her relatives took her to a hospital. The preceding day she had mistakenly defecated in a trash can, thinking she was in her bathroom.
>
> The woman was "cleared medically." She was given a diagnosis of "acute grief reaction," and admitted to the psychiatric service. She was unable to recall one of three items after 5 minutes. Also, she was found to have a peculiar yellow coloring of the sclerae of her eyes. (Weissberg, 1979)

This woman had a known history of chronic liver disease related to alcoholism. Her liver disease put her at risk for organic mental disorder. Subsequent laboratory studies confirmed that she had contracted viral hepatitis, thereby compromising her already debilitated liver to the extent that she went into hepatic (liver) failure. This was the cause of her symptoms. Her history of alcoholism and chronic liver disease should have served as important alerting clues to the true nature of her problem.

Use of Drugs

Psychoactive chemicals create an elaborate array of mental and emotional changes that can be pleasurable, frightening, or bizarre. Adverse reactions to drugs are the number one cause of organic mental disorder. Furthermore, with certain substances, addiction can ensue. If the person's drug supply is then interrupted, severe withdrawal characterized by anxiety, confusion, or even psychosis occurs. Although wild, agitated delirium is easily recognized, drug reactions can be much more subtle in their presentation.

In addition to toxic effects, excessive use of drugs (including alcohol) predisposes a person to a myriad of medical problems as well as accidents, particularly related to driving.

The clinician should not overlook the fact that prescription and over-the-counter medications are *drugs*. Increasingly, these substances account for organic mental disorders; and, in psychiatry the same medications used for treatment produce their own "psychiatric symptoms."

Persons taking over-the-counter drugs sometimes do not consider them medications. They may unknowingly mislead the clinician by denying the use of medications even though they are taking self-prescribed preparations, some of which have powerful "mind-bending" effects.

> For a period of two months, he had slept infrequently. Sometimes he would work two consecutive shifts, one for pay, the other for free. He would throw himself feverishly into whatever he was doing. An example was bowling. He had been known to bowl 50 games uninterrupted! He often became impatient, resetting the pins if he did not score a strike with the first ball.
>
> As they watched their son overspend his income and squander his savings, the parents of this 23-year-old man became concerned. On the day prior to his hospitalization, he disrobed in front of his mother and tried to climb into a small wash basin. After becoming agitated when his father restrained him, he was taken to the hospital.
>
> The young man was described as oriented but with obvious paranoid delusions. There was no memory impairment or hallucinations. He denied using drugs. (Sayed, 1976)

It was determined that this man had recently experienced an acne-like rash. This subtle clue led to a laboratory finding of "bromide toxicity." Within a week the man's normal behavior had returned. Upon further questioning, he related that he had been ingesting on a daily basis a bromide preparation sold over-the-counter.

The clinician should inquire routinely about drugs and medications. This aspect of history-taking, whenever possible, should involve a secondary source whenever there is initial evidence of a problem. Persons who abuse drugs are unreliable reporters.

There is another aspect of drugs to consider. While many persons get into difficulty abusing drugs, others have problems because they do *not* take drugs. For certain persons, medications are essential. If they are not taken with regularity, the person becomes seriously ill, such as happens in diabetes, severe hypertension, heart failure, asthma, hypothyroidism, and many other conditions. Despite the risks involved, for one reason or another, patients often stop taking medications on their own. This can cause psychological masquerade.

> Her negative feelings about the Immigration and Naturalization Service began to get out of hand. She was a 36-year-old Mexican woman, married for ten years and described by her husband as a normal housewife. There was no history of psychiatric problems, until she required hospitalization following a week of sleepless agitation and psychotic thinking. She became frightened and suspicious of cars and people, particularly agents of the INS whom she felt were stalking her. In the hospital she expressed the belief that someone was impersonating her sister in order to arrange her own murder.
>
> She appeared depressed. Her face was expressionless. Her movements were slow, but she was fully oriented and had no memory problem.
>
> It was learned that nine years previously, she had been found to have hypothyroidism. A daily thyroid supplement (levothyroixine sodium, 15 mg per day) was prescribed. Two months prior to her hospitalization, she had stopped taking it. Her hypothyroid problem was confirmed by laboratory tests. Within 11 days of restarting thyroid hormone, the woman's mental status had returned to normal. (Santiago, Stoker, Beigel, Yost, & Spencer, 1987)

Failure to take necessary medication can have serious psychological consequences. (Incidentally, this is an interesting clinical example of Capgras' syndrome, a delusional condition in which the afflicted person believes that a loved one has been mysteriously replaced by an identical double. This syndrome is sometimes stress-related, but also has been described in a number of organic disorders.)

The role of drugs and medications in producing organic mental disorders is so extensive that I have devoted a later chapter exclusively to this subject.

PRESUMPTIVE CLUES

The clues discussed in this section are so often associated with organic mental disorders that when detected in the presence of psychological symptoms, organic mental disorders should be assumed until proven otherwise.

Head Injury

Head injury always raises the specter of a neurological condition. Head trauma sometimes causes increased pressure within the brain. Most cases produce symptoms readily recognized as neurological deficits and thus do not characteristically masquerade.

A major exception is seen in alcoholics, where acute neurological symptoms may be mistaken for signs of drunkenness. The inebriated person may pass out while standing upright or driving a car and sustain a traumatic head injury. Upon arousing, the person may be unable to describe the injury or the resulting symptoms and may be written off as "just another drunk."

In emergency settings, clinicians should always look for obvious signs of recent head trauma, such as facial lacerations, broken teeth, dried blood around the ear, or an unexplained lump on the head, particularly if the person is intoxicated.

In some cases of head injury, symptoms are slow to evolve and may be restricted to subtle changes in personality or vague complaints of headache. Automobile accidents frequently cause head injury, even though no external evidence may be seen and the person may not report a loss of consciousness. Sometimes direct questions such as "Have you been in a recent automobile accident or otherwise injured?" will bring to light instances of injury that otherwise would go unacknowledged.

Change in Headache Pattern

A recent *change* in a person's headache pattern should be thoroughly evaluated medically. Headache is a relatively common experience among adults. Typically there is a well-established pattern of onset and distribution of pain, often in response to various life stresses. The person comes to know this symptom as a stress reaction, relieved by lowering the stress level or by simple treatment such as taking aspirin. When a person seeking help from a therapist or counselor spontaneously complains of a *different kind of headache*, the clinician should pay particular attention.

Headache can be a symptom of serious brain diseases, particularly infections, brain tumors, and subdural hematomas. One researcher has estimated that approximately 60% of persons with brain tumors have associated headaches. Headache is the *initial* manifestation of brain tumor in one out of five cases! The percentage for subdural hematoma is even higher. Additionaly, as we shall discuss in Chapter 7, the type of headache classically associated with brain tumor has a characteristic pattern with which all clinicians should be familiar.

In addition to inquiring about a change in headache pattern, the clinician should also be sensitive to nonverbal clues. Once again, this is especially important when dealing with intoxicated persons and with persons who are confused, drowsy, or psychotic. The person may intermittently pull at his ear or hold his head in his hands. These gestures may be the only evidence of headache.

The following case illustrates how easily headache can be neglected when it is associated with psychological symptoms.

> A young man in his early twenties, hyperactive and abusively threatening violence, was evaluated in an emergency room.
>
> His wife said that on the previous day he had started complaining of a severe headache for which he was seen by his family physician and treated with a "pain shot." But the headache persisted. Later, at home, the man abruptly started screaming and attacked both his wife and children. The Fire Department was summoned, and he was taken to the hospital.
>
> He appeared in good physical health but was incoherent. Without provocation, he would become wild, screaming at other people. He was treated with an antipsychotic medication and admitted as a case of functional psychosis (schizophrenia).
>
> Over the next 24 hours, the young man became increasingly drowsy and developed fever and a stiff neck. Special neurological studies showed meningoencephalitis, an infection of the brain and its coverings. Fortunately, aggressive antibiotic therapy was successful. There were no residual effects. (Sandler, 1975)

Visual Disturbances

Any visual problem of recent onset suggests the possibility of organic disorder. The clinician should be particularly alert to complaints or evidence of double vision or partial visual loss.

Eye movement is the product of complex muscle coordination, requiring balanced input from several different nerves. The three cranial nerves that control eye movement extend for varying lengths from their points of origin in the brain to their connections with the muscles of the eyes. Consequently, they are susceptible to encroachment by expanding brain masses or injury from certain degenerative diseases. When these nerves are compromised, the fine movement of the eyes is disrupted. To the observer, the eyes may appear out of line or crossed. Since the muscle imbalance leads to image formation on slightly different areas of each retina, the person will complain of "seeing double."

The visual pathways from the retina to the occipital cortex (and surrounding associative areas) also can be interrupted by various brain diseases. In some instances, the visual disturbance may be so subtle that the person fails to notice. Nevertheless, the person may be left with a "hole" in his sight that becomes apparent only after a series of unexplained accidents, such as bumping into doorways or scraping the car when driving into narrow parking spaces. This is because the person is unable to detect objects in certain parts of the visual fields, right or left depending on where the brain disorder is located.

In other cases the person will be fully aware of a visual problem. When this occurs in association with psychological symptoms, an organic mental disorder should be considered.

Speech Deficits

Speech deficits can be categorized roughly into two groups: problems in the mechanical production of speech sounds and problems in appropriate word usage.

Difficulty articulating words is called *dysarthria*. The most common cause is drug or alcohol intoxication. The person's speech is slurred and "thick," sometimes to the extent of being impossible to understand. Although an observant clinician should not make this error, dysarthric speech can be mistaken for psychotic language. The speech of persons in the throes of functional psychosis, although strange in its content, usually is mechanically intact. It is not dysarthric.

In contrast to dysarthria, aphasia is the loss of word comprehension and proper word usage. In one form, known as *nonfluent aphasia*, in addition to the person's having difficulty finding the right word, the natural flow and rhythm of speech is lost. Characteristically, the person uses mainly verbs and nouns, with a scarcity of modifiers or connecting words. Nonfluent aphasia frequently results from a stroke which also leaves the person with a restriction in movement on one side of the body (usually the right side); for this reason, it seldom presents as a psychological masquerade, because it is readily identifiable as a neurological condition.

Not so, however, with, *fluent aphasia*, which can easily be mistaken for a psychiatric problem. In this condition, the person has no difficulty articulating words. The speech is smooth and naturally rhythmic, but the person has great difficulty finding the correct words and arranging them so that they communicate the desired meaning. When closely examined, the person's speech has little substantive content. It is filled with incorrect, inappropriate, or even made-up words.

The individual with fluent aphasia, surprisingly, often seems unaware that anything is wrong. The person may talk around the word that cannot be mobilized. For example, in trying to say "key," the person might come up with "what you unlock the door with"; or, in referring to a spoon, "a handle with a little cup on it."

Word substitution may be used, so "hammer" is used for the related word "nail," or "fork" for "knife." Word substitutions may be made on the basis of similar sounds. "Spoot" might be used for "spoon" or "heart" for "hard." Sometimes the process seems almost random, as in one writer's report of a patient who referred to his thumb as an "Argentinean rifle" (Geschwind, 1971). Prepositions and other connecting words are especially troublesome. This causes rough grammatic transitions, difficult to follow.

One of the most confusing variations of fluent aphasia is the prominent use of artificial words known as "neologisms." These fabricated words sound bizarre; they are easily mistaken for psychotic speech. The difference is that, while the psychotic person periodically uses strange words, there is generally no ongoing difficulty with descriptive language. For the aphasic, the routine use of language is problematic.

The most common form of fluent aphasia is limited to the naming of well-known objects, a condition called *anomia*. The person has difficulty coming up with common names. Also, if asked to list various items in a class—such as animals or vegetables—the person will have considerable difficulty. Anomia may occur alone or in combination with other forms of aphasia. It is important to recognize because it is a symptom found in a number of neurological disorders.

> Dr. Bruce Dobkin, a Los Angeles neurologist and writer, in an article entitled "Ironman," recounts an exchange between himself and an athlete who had become aphasic following a cerebral hemorrhage. The 40-year-old man, upon completing an eight-mile run, developed a severe headache. He tried to go to work the next day, but the pain was incapacitating. Afterwards, he recounted the details for Dr. Dobkin.

> PATIENT: "I got home and back into bed. My wife called again when it was dark, and told me to call the blotcher."
> DOCTOR: "Blotcher?"
> PATIENT: "Ah, you know, the one like you. I mean, the. . . ."
> DOCTOR: "Doctor?"
> PATIENT: "Yeah, that's it."

> Later on, the same patient, speaking of his physical limitations, commented: "I guess I have some *laminations*." (Dobkin, 1988)

When a person with aphasia is unable to communicate what he wants to say, he becomes frustrated, raising his voice so as to be understood. Add to this a smattering of neologisms plus a few awkward expressions and you have a worthy challenge for any clinician to recognize this psychological masquerade.

Differentiation of aphasia from psychiatric symptoms requires an active suspicion and careful listening. One researcher put it this way: "The acute onset of abnormal speech in a middle-aged person is . . . almost invariably diagnostic of a fluent (receptive) aphasia (Geschwind, 1971). Any evidence of a mechanical defect (such as slurred or garbled speech) or of trouble communicating simple facts or naming common objects should be considered a possible neurological problem.

This next case history illustrates the last three presumptive clues we have considered: change in headache pattern, visual disturbances, and speech deficits.

A middle-aged man required restraints made from heavy fish netting to control his violent, explosive behavior. As he was being admitted to the hospital, he was observed to snarl, show his teeth, and lash out at bystanders.

Previously in the day, for no apparent reason, he had attacked his wife with a butcher knife. When the police arrived at his home, the man was observed to have severely garbled speech.

Over the past several months, he had undergone a striking personality change and had complained of blurred vision and severe headaches.

He was found to have a large, right frontal lobe tumor extending into the temporal area as well. After the surgical removal, his symptoms disappeared, allowing him to resume his job as a night watchman. (Mark & Ervin, 1970)

Abnormal Body Movements

Many clinicians fail to appreciate the close connection between abnormal body movements and organic mental disorders.

Take simple, ordinary walking. This basic human skill is disturbed in a number of conditions that cause psychological masquerades. Unsteadiness is an important clue to drug and alcohol intoxication. When manifest by gross staggering, the clinical detection is easy; but, when the person compensates by walking with a wider-based gait and moving slowly and more deliberately, clinical recognition becomes more difficult.

Syphilis of the brain, pernicious anemia (vitamin B_{12} deficiency) alcoholism, and a number of other organic disorders produce psychological symptoms in combination with disturbances in walking. Normal pressure hydrocephalus, a condition usually commencing in mid-life, causes declining mental ability (usually with depression), loss of bladder control, and a peculiar disturbance in walking. The person has difficulty initiating each step. The feet seem stuck to the floor, hence the term *magnetic gait.*

Every clinician should develop a sense of what constitutes normal walking: how the arms swing, how far apart the feet are, the relative length of normal striding. Consequently, on the basis of a brief observation, aberrations in walking should be obvious. In the interview situation, this is easily and unobtrusively accomplished by watching a person enter and leave the office.

Other kinds of abnormal movements also serve as indicators of psychological masquerade. Persons with Parkinson's disease experience depression and emotional lability along with a characteristic tremor of the hands, sometimes described as "pill-rolling" movements. Huntington's chorea causes poor impulse control and eventually may manifest as violence and psychosis. A hallmark of this condition is *spastic jerking* and *twitching* of various muscles throughout the body, particularly in the extremities and the trunk. In Wilson's disease, (a disorder of copper metabolism) tremor, spasms, and dysarthria may accompany mania, depression, or schizoaffective psychosis.

The combination of psychological symptoms and abnormal movements is not as surprising as it may seem. Brain areas active in motor coordination and emotional elaboration both contain high concentrations of the same neurotransmitter, dopamine. It is presumed that disturbances in this chemical in relation to other neurotransmitters simultaneously produce abnormal movements and psychological symptoms. Tremors, tics, twitches, jerking movements, and difficulty walking should not be overlooked by the clinician. They are often the main clues to organic mental disorder.

Sustained Deviations in Vital Signs

Vital signs refer collectively to heart rate, blood pressure, respiratory rate, and temperature. These four measures reflect the physiological integrity of the body. Generally, they remain within relatively narrow ranges. With physical stress or anxiety, significant deviations in heart rate, blood pressure, temperature, or respirations occur temporarily; but, as a general rule, when one or more of these vital signs remains abnormal for a period of several hours or more, organic disease should be suspected.

In some instances, particularly when drugs are involved, a change in vital signs may be the *only* indicator of organicity. Vital sign determinations are not highly technical measurements, and their use as *screening measures* does not necessarily require medical expertise. I am not suggesting that nonmedical professionals assume primary responsibility for vital sign measurements. They should, however, make use of this valuable source of information when it is available and also request it when appropriate.

TABLE 5.1 Vital Sign Values

For critical assessment screening

Heart Rate:	50–100/minute
Blood Pressure:	90–160 (systolic)
	50–95 (diastolic)
Respirations:	6–20/minute
Temperature (oral):	96°F. (35.6°C) – 100° F. (37.8°C)

In Table 5.1 numerical values are listed that can be used by the clinician for detecting vital sign deviations. Determinations *outside* these ranges (if found in the absence of stress) should be considered pathological.

Following two days of confusion, disorientation, and the obsessive thought that he had a transistor radio in his head, a young man was admitted to the emergency ward.

He appeared "delirious." His memory for recent events was obviously impaired. Measurements of his vital signs were recorded: blood pressure— 140/100, pulse—120, and rectal temperature—100.2° F. His pupils were widely dilated and did not contract in response to light.

Despite these abnormal findings, the initial clinical impression was that this man was experiencing psychotic excitement. Treatment with intramuscular haloperidol, however, had no effect.

Three hours later, the young man's family brought in an empty pill bottle that had contained amitriptyline (Elavil®). This discovery, combined with the man's clinical appearance and abnormal vital signs, led to a diagnosis of anticholinergic psychosis. Physostigmine was given and within 45 minutes the delirium had cleared, only to return after two and a half hours, when the short-acting drug had worn off. Repeated treatments, however, produced complete resolution. He was discharged 36 hours later, fully recovered. (Grancher & Baldessarini, 1975)

A clinician oblivious to this patient's abnormal vital signs might have held to the mistaken idea that this was a functional psychotic episode.

(A word of caution about vital signs. These measures are sometimes hastily taken and recorded. When a significant deviation is discovered, the first course of action should be to repeat the measure. This simple rule can save considerable time and energy directed at false findings.)

Changes in Consciousness

Consciousness is a person's state of alertness and general awareness. Three changes in consciousness should always suggest organic dysfunction. They are: excessive sleepiness, lapses, and loss of consciousness.

Excessive sleepiness is associated with many brain disorders. The clinical history often includes falling asleep in the middle of the day, even during the course of conversation. The person may frequently fall asleep while working. Typically, the problem is dramatically magnified by even small amounts of alcohol or tranquilizers.

A lapse in consciousness is a momentary break in a person's awareness. There may be no memory of such lapses; thus, the person (particularly in cases where the lapses are quite brief) may be unaware of the problem. When observed by the clinician, lapses can be mistaken for blocking, a symptom seen in schizophenia. The person may suddenly for no apparent reason cease talking, only to resume after a momentary pause as though nothing had happened. More often than not, true lapses indicate seizure activity arising deep in the brain.

> The family physician of a 26-year-old man referred him with the brief notation that he was "psychotic and needed hospitalization."
>
> While at work that day, the man thought he smelled acetylene gas. Concerned about a possible explosion, he crawled out on the roof of his shop to investigate. What he "found" was unexpected. He saw "tanks of gas" pouring over into the air conditioning system. He immediately called the local police and fire departments, but when they arrived, they found nothing. The man was referred to his physician and then to the hospital.
>
> There was no history of mental illness or drug use. On mental status examination, the man appeared normal without disorientation, delusions, or hallucinations. Further questioning, however, revealed a history of short lapses in consciousness, one of which had resulted in an automobile accident. (Lawall, 1976)

This man was having seizures, confirmed by an electroencephalogram which recorded "random sharp spikes" over the left temporal lobe area. The final diagnosis was temporal lobe epilepsy.

Fainting spells or any other form of loss of consciousness should receive a thorough medical examination without exception. One would think that unexplained loss of consciousness invariably would raise the suspicion of neurological disorder, but as the next case illustrates, this is not always true.

> While on business in another country, an atomic physicist began to have paranoid thoughts of people plotting to steal atomic secrets from him. Within

a short while the seriousness of his condition became obvious. He was quickly returned home, where he was diagnosed as schizophrenic and hospitalized for psychiatric treatment.

After his release several months later, he suffered a loss of consciousness with a grand mal seizure. Still, his psychiatrist, firmly convinced that the man was experiencing a schizophrenic break, dismissed the possibility of an organic mental disorder. Only after he complained of a severe, unrelenting headache was he referred for neurological studies. He was found to have a highly malignant brain tumor invading the temporal lobe. (Geschwind, 1975)

SPECIAL CLINICAL TESTING

We have considered five alerting clues and eight presumptive clues (including symptoms of brain syndrome) important to the clinical recognition of psychological masquerade. These clinical clues are the clinician's basic keys to unmasking psychological masquerade. There will be situations, however, where the evidence is equivocal or only suggestive, leaving the clinician undecided. In such instances, the following three special tests may provide helpful information. These three tests are simple in design and can be administered in a brief period, ordinarily in less than 10 minutes (for all three). If any of the three are positive, the clinician should consider this presumptive evidence of an organic mental problem. When *negative*, however, these tests should not be construed as definitive evidence against organicity. They are unquantitated tests and in no way substitute for more sophisticated neuropsychological testing.

Write-a-Sentence Test

Despite the appearance of simplicity, the task of writing a sentence requires highly complex brain–eye–muscle interaction. The Write-a-Sentence Test is a particularly sensitive indicator of global brain dysfunction and typically shows improvement parallelling a person's recovery (Chidru & Geschwind 1972).

The test is administered by giving the following verbal instructions: "Write the sentence which I give you as neatly and legibly as you can. The sentence is: "Men and women have equal rights but different needs."

This sentence should be slowly stated *twice* to ensure that the person adequately registers it. The person should be provided with lined paper and a pencil. (Of course, if there is a language preferred to English, the sentence should be given in that language.)

When the person has completed the sentence or at the end of two minutes, whichever happens first, the sentence should be reviewed for the following deficits: completion; clumsily formed letters; duplication of certain writing strokes, particularly in letters such as m or w improper alignment of letters, with displacement either upward or downward from the line. Spelling errors, use of nonexistent words (neologisms); word deletions or word repetitions. Detailed, microscopic analysis should not be employed. Look for obvious errors as a basis for calling the test positive.

Draw-a-Clock Test

This test requires that a person handle spatial relationships, simple number sequences, writing numbers, and time representation (see Figure 5.1). The task is not dependent on verbal skills and therefore is subject to relatively little cultural distortion. Although a simple task for most adults of normal intelligence, the Draw-a-Clock Test may prove highly problematic for a person with an organic brain disorder.

The test is given by providing the person with a previously printed circle, approximately 3 inches in diameter. (It is a good idea to have a supply of these printed circles available in the clinic setting.) The person is given a pencil and instructed to enter the appropriate numbers as they ordinarily appear on the face of a clock and then to draw the hands so that the time shown is 10 minutes past 10 o'clock.

When the person has completed the task or at the end of two minutes, whichever comes first, the construction should be reviewed with the following facts in mind. Persons with organic brain disease (associative areas) may displace the numbers on the clock so that they fall outside the circle or gravitate toward the center. Crowding, repeating, or deleting numbers may also occur, as well as a rotation of the numbers so that 12 no longer appears at the top. Sometimes the person will draw the hands of the clock so that they are displaced from the center of the circle or represent an incorrect time (Robbins & Stern, 1976).

If a person is unable to complete this test without obvious errors, it should be considered presumptive evidence of an organic disorder. Further evaluation is indicated.

Copy-a-Three-Dimensional-Figure Test

This is a test of spatial appreciation. Adequate performance depends on the integrity of various associative areas of the brain. Since these areas are extensive in size and relatively silent with respect to motor movement and

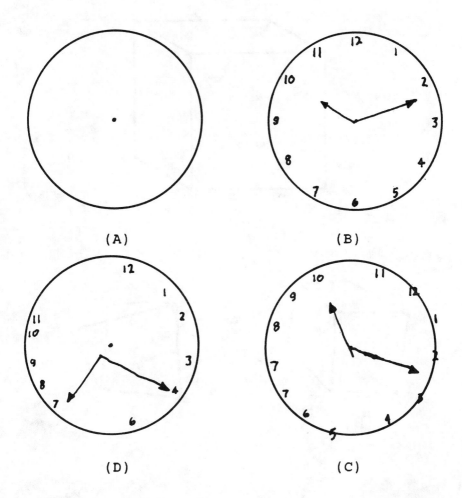

FIGURE 5.1 Draw-a-Clock test. **A:** Printed circle with dot in center. **B:** Adequate reproduction. **C:** Displacement and rotation of numbers; repetition of a number (7). **D:** Crowding; displacement of hands; deletion of a number (5); incorrect time.

sensory perception, this simple constructional test can be a critical screening device for organic dysfunction which might otherwise go undetected.

The test is administered by giving the person a previously printed, three-dimensional figure such as a cube. He is instructed to copy the figure in a space provided just below the printed version. When the person has completed the task or at the end of two minutes, whichever comes first, the construction is reviewed (see Figure 5.2).

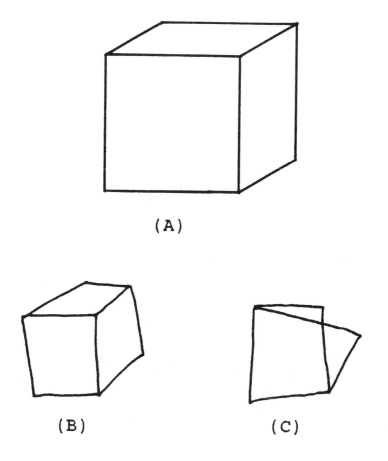

(A)

(B)   **(C)**

FIGURE 5.2 Copy-a-Three-Dimensional-Figure test. **A:** Printed cube which client copys. **B:** Adequate reproduction. **C:** Inadequate reproduction.

Evaluation of this test consists of judging whether or not the person has been able to reproduce the three-dimensional effect. If the reproduced figure is flat and two-dimensional in appearance, the test is positive.

In the preceding two chapters we have discussed crucial clinical clues to masquerading organic conditions. Alerting clues should sensitize the clinician. In turn, the identification of any one of several presumptive clues demands further medical evaluation. Sometimes these clues will be misleading in that no organicity will be found. In a significant number of cases, however, an underlying organic disorder will be detected. Persistent searching for these clues provides the clinician with a sound approach to psychological masquerade.

We have not reviewed the use of specialized tests such as the CAT scan, EEG, and lumbar puncture. While these are potent assessment tools, they fall within the domain of medical specialists. They are more appropriate as second-line tests, used to arrive at specific neurological diagnoses. Although, to be sure, these procedures are an important part of the workup for organic mental disorder, our focus in this book is on nonmedical clinical assessment.

In the next chapter, we will look at how the clinician integrates the search for psychological masquerade into the basic clinical interview.

REFERENCES

Carlson, R. (1977). Frontal lobe lesions masquerading as psychiatric disturbances. *Canadian Psychiatric Association Journal, 22,* 315–318.

Chidru, F., & Geschwind, N. (1972). Writing disturbances in acute confusional states. *Neuropsychological, 10,* 343–353.

Dobkin, B. (1988, September 4). The Ironman. *The New York Times Magazine,* pp. 40–41.

Geschwind, N. (1971). Current concepts: aphasia. *New England Journal of Medicine, 284,* 654–657.

Geschwind, N. (1975). In F. Benson & D. Blumer (Eds.), *Psychiatric aspects of neurological disease,* volume 7. New York: Grune and Stratton.

Grancher, R., & Baldessarini, R. (1975). Physostigmine. *Archives of General Psychiatry, 32,* 375–380.

Lawall, J. (1976). Psychiatric presentations of seizure disorders. *Amrican Journal of Psychiatry, 133,* 321–323.

Mark, V., & Ervin, F. (1970). *Violence in the brain.* New York, Harper and Row.

Robbins, E., & Stern, M. (1976). Assessment of psychiatric emergencies. In R. Glick, A. Meyerson, E. Robbins, and J. Talbott *Psychiatric emergencies,* (9–48). New York: Grune and Stratton.

Sandler, N. (1975). A case of meningitis admitted as schizophrenia. *Journal of the Kentucky Medical Association, 73,* 25–26.

Santiago, J., Stoker, D., Beigel, A., Yost, D., & Spencer, P. (1987). Capgras' Syndrome in a Myxedema patient. *Hospital and Community Psychiatry, 38,* 199–201.

Sayed, J. (1971). Mania and bromism: a case report and a look at the future, *American Journal of Psychiatry, 133,* 228–229.

Waggoner, R., & Bagohi, B. (1954). Initial masking of organic brain changes by psychic symptoms. *American Journal of Psychiatry, 110,* 904–910.

Weissberg, M. (1979). Emergency room medical clearance: an educational problem. *American Journal of Psychiatry, 136,* 787–790.

Chapter 6

Looking for Psychological Masquerade in the Clinical Setting

Practice and thought might gradually forge many an art.   —*Virgil*

Having read through the previous chapter, the reader may feel over-whelmed by the list of assessment factors. So this is an appropriate point to pause, take a breath, and consider the nuts and bolts of looking for psychological masquerade in the clinical setting. It's not as onerous a task as at first it may appear to be.

A complete check list is provided in Table 6.1. The clinician should resist the tendency to run through this list as a separate part of the interview. Although such an approach may prove easier initially, in the long run it is much more intrusive than an approach which weaves these questions into the overall interview. With practice, your own natural style will prevail. Looking for psychological masquerade will become second nature requiring a surprisingly small amount of extra interview time.

In Figure 6.1, I have indicated where (in the ordinary course of an inter-view) various issues typically will be addressed. In a clinical setting, the per-son's age (and sometimes vital signs) may be noted on the admission form or in the patient's record. The first part of an interview will focus on the chief complaint and stresses in the person's life. It is also quite natural to inquire early about a history of similar symptoms.

Throughout the interview, the clinician should be on the lookout for changes in consciousness, abnormal body movements, speech deficits, and evidence of brain syndrome. Evidence may also turn up in the person's history; this is particularly true of changes in consciousness. Remaining questions can be naturally woven into the interview. If indicated, the special

TABLE 6.1 Clues to Psychological Masquerade

Alerting clues
1. No history of similar symptoms
2. No readily identifiable cause
3. Age 55 or older
4. Coexistence of chronic disease
5. Use of drugs

Presumptive clues
6. Brain syndrome (one or more core deficits)
→ Disorientation
→ Recent memory impairment
→ Diminshed reasoning
→ Sensory indiscrimination
7. Head injury
8. Change in headache pattern
9. Visual disturbances
10. Speech deficits
11. Abnormal body movements
12. Sustained deviations in vital signs
13. Changes in consciousness
14. Special tests
→ Write-a-Sentence
→ Draw-a-Clock
→ Copy-a-Three-Dimensional-Figure

construction tests can be administered toward the end, when their appropriateness can better be determined.

HYPOTHETICAL CASES

As a way of reviewing these guidelines, let's consider a hypothetical case. You are about to see a new patient. The week prior he has arranged for an appointment. This is your first meeting. The receptionist calls your office, announcing that Mr. B has arrived. You go to meet him in the waiting area and, after introducing yourself, escort him back to your office. You are both seated. The information sheet says that he is a 45-year-old automobile salesman.

By this time—even though the formal interview has yet to begin—you should have made several pertinent observations. You have had an oppor-

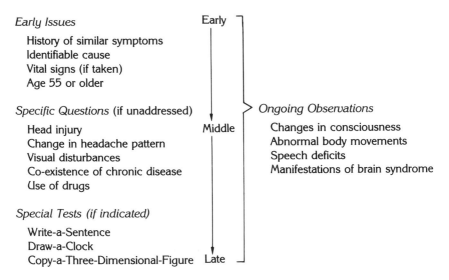

FIGURE 6.1 Course of the interview.

tunity to observe the man's general appearance and dress as well as the way he walks. Is there anything unusual about his general appearance? Is his shirt wrong-side-out? Does he have difficulty walking? Positive answers to these questions might suggest neurological deficits. The point is this: even before you ask the first question, observations pertinent to screening for psychological masquerade should have been made.

You might start the interview with the question, "What brings you here?" As the individual tells his story, he may relate a history of similar symptoms or reveal a stressful life situation. If this information is not spontaneously touched on, you will want to insert specific inquiries at appropriate junctures. For example, in our hypothetical case, the man states that he has been feeling depressed. The interview might then proceed as follows:

INTERVIEWER: "In the past, have you ever been depressed the way you are now?"

CLIENT: "Well, I have felt blue at times, a little down . . . but never like this. I don't want to do anything. I avoid friends. Nothing seems to mean much anymore."

You have pretty well established that the man has no prior history of the kind of depression he now is experiencing.

As the interview progresses, you continuously observe for shifts in consciousness, abnormal body movements, and speech deficits. Each of these symptoms can manifest episodically during the course of the interview and may be overlooked unless you are actively watching. This does not require a sustained, intense focus of attention, but more of a heightened suspicion, watching "out of the corner of one's eye," so to speak.

So, relatively early into the interview, you are unobtrusively collecting information pertinent to detecting psychological masquerade. As the patient proceeds with his story, essential pieces of information are volunteered. As this occurs, you should note it, thereby avoiding the need for redundant questions.

Our hypothetical patient elaborates about his depression by describing how nothing seems to be going right. Sales are down. His car has been in the shop twice in the last 3 weeks. One of his children has had a "brush with the law," and he has been having "a bitch of a headache" for the past 2 days. While describing situational events, he has mentioned an unexpected symptom—headache. It is incumbent on you to explore this "red-flag" complaint.

INTERVIEWER: "About this headache you have been having, describe it for me."
CLIENT: "Oh, it's the kind I always get; right in the back of my neck. If I take three aspirin early enough, I can usually nip it in the bud; otherwise, it will go on for most of the day. I've had these things off and on for 30 years. My doctor never has found anything wrong. I think it's just stress."
INTERVIEWER: "Is there anything *different* about your headache this time?"
CLIENT: "No, it's the same. Every damn time, just like clockwork, when I get loaded down with pressures: headache time!"

Through this brief exchange, you have confirmed that the client has had a headache with which he has become quite familiar over the years. It is not a new headache pattern, and unless it should persist beyond its typical duration, it would *not* constitute presumptive evidence for an organic mental disorder.

If by midway in the interview certain questions have not been addressed, you will want to look for a natural transition and inquire specifically about them.

INTERVIEWER: "Mr. B, I want to ask you a few questions about your general health that might possibly have a bearing on the way you are feeling. Have you had any recent head injury?"
CLIENT: "No."
INTERVIEWER: "Has your vision changed? Have you been having trouble seeing? Have you had double vision?"
CLIENT: "No, I haven't had anything like that."

INTERVIEWER: "What about medical problems?"

CLIENT: "My doctor tells me I have bronchitis. I know I smoke too much."

INTERVIEWER: "Do you take medications, either prescribed or those you get for yourself at the drug store?"

CLIENT: "No."

INTERVIEWER: "No medications for your lung problems? None at all?"

CLIENT: "Well, I use aspirin and sometimes I take something for heartburn, but I don't use either one of them very often."

INTERVIEWER: "How about alcohol or other drugs? How much do you use?"

CLIENT: "I have a cocktail just about every evening and sometimes a beer or two on weekends. I don't use any kind of drugs."

INTERVIEWER: "Has a doctor ever told you something was wrong with your heart, your blood pressure, or the way you breathe?"

CLIENT: "No. Even with all my smoking, every time my doctor checks me, he says everything is pretty good."

This short series of questions probably would take less than two minutes. From the answers provided by our hypothetical patient, the only item that would be remotely suggestive of psychological masquerade is the possibility of chronic lung disease. Along with the fact that the man has apparently never before experienced a significant depression, it serves as an alerting clue.

Let us assume, in this case, that no presumptive clues are identified. You have been particularly alert for evidence of brain syndrome. There is none. He is obviously aware of the time and where he is. The manner in which he goes about telling his story demonstrates that he is completely alert. At one point in the interview you test his recent memory by giving him three objects to remember; and, after 5 minutes he recalls them all. Throughout the interview you have looked for changes in consciousness. You have seen nothing even remotely suspicious.

If his vital signs are noted in the chart, you might check to confirm that they are normal. If during the interview you have heard something that makes you suspicious of the man's statement about his drug and alcohol use, you might return to this with more insistent questioning; or, better still, if his spouse is waiting outside, you might want to pose the same question to her.

Assume no further evidence is detected. You are left with a middle-aged man whose life situation is compatible with feeling depressed, and who has never before had this problem. He may have chronic bronchitis for which, however, he requires no medication. Organic mental disorder is an unlikely possibility. Even so, if you are still concerned about the possibility of psychological masquerade, you could administer the three special construction tests. Let's assume that this is done, and our hypothetical patient performs all of them quickly and without error.

At this juncture, you proceed to characterize the man's depressed mood as a psychological reaction, realizing, nevertheless, that later on presumptive evidence for an organic mental disorder could still turn up. The process of looking for psychological masquerade is never complete. Clinicians should maintain an ongoing vigil for relevant clues. They pop up at the strangest times.

Consider a second hypothetical case. A woman, age 45, is brought by her husband for psychological assessment. On the intake form—which you are handed when the woman, escorted by her husband, enters your office—is listed the chief complaint: "Nervousness." The woman's husband immediately takes over the interview, relating how his wife has been hospitalized on two previous occasions for manic behavior. Each time she has gradually become more and more agitated, going without sleep, and talking in nonstop fashion. As the husband tells her story, the woman seems anxious. You politely interrupt, saying that you would like to hear from his wife; but, when you ask her what seems to be the problem, she is hesitant to talk. Finally, when she does so, she is unable to tell a coherent story. As you attempt to clarify the problem by questioning her, she becomes frustrated and begins to cry. Her husband breaks in, insisting that she be hospitalized since she is "obviously having another manic attack." But when you ask him to describe how this current episode started, he appears perplexed, and admits that, actually, it was quite different from her other attacks. All of a sudden, the preceding day, she began to talk "crazy."

By this time, you have been able to observe for changes in consciousness and abnormal body movements. There have been none. The woman appears oriented. There is no evidence that she is experiencing illusions or hallucinations. When you check her recent memory, she recalls three items, although she eventually has to point to a book (the three item), appearing to have difficulty getting the word out. You proceed to ask her specifically about recent head injury, changes in headache, visual problems, chronic disease and drug/alcohol use. She starts to answer, but her husband breaks in and answers for her. Other than for her irregular use of a laxative and infrequent drinking on weekends, all questions are answered negatively.

You can't quite put your finger on it, but something doesn't add up. You decide to administer the three special tests. The woman has no trouble reproducing the stated time on a printed clock face or copying the three-dimensional figure. She does, however, have difficulty writing the sentence you have given her. She has left out a word and given a strange spelling to a second word. As you are discussing this with her, you realize that she is having trouble understanding what you are asking her. You check this out by having her name a few common objects in your office. She is unable to identify several of them. Asked to name ten animals, she comes up with only three: dog, cat, and cow.

This woman has a notable speech deficit, probably aphasic in nature. You now have presumptive evidence for organicity; evidence that necessitates further medical evaluation.

You inform the patient and her husband that you suspect her problem is not another manic attack; she needs further evaluation which you can arrange for her that same afternoon.

In a case where presumptive evidence for psychological masquerade is uncovered, the clinician should not prematurely communicate his suspicion to the patient. Instead, the person should be told of the need for further evaluation and an appropriate referral arranged as soon as possible. It is important that the referral be followed up to ensure that the evaluation does take place. Of course, this will also provide the clinician with instructive feedback.

SELF-TEST

Before proceeding to the next chapter, let's see how well you have mastered the various clues to psychological masquerade. On the following pages you will find five case histories. Try reading them and identifying any evidence of organic mental disorder. Following each history, you will find an explanation and a discussion of specific clues.

CASE HISTORY #1: SENDING A MESSAGE

A 25-year-old college student was escorted by a friend to the emergency room of a large, city hospital. The friend related that the man's wife, arriving at home after work, had found her husband acting strangely, stumbling about the apartment, alternately laughing and crying, incoherent at times.

When examined, the patient mumbled without making sense and would not respond to direct questions. Periodically he bent down close to the floor, as though trying to pick up something. Over the course of several hours, his condition fluctuated from passive withdrawal to combative agitation. His pupils were widely dilated.

Later, the man's wife arrived at the hospital and provided further information. She said that her husband was not a drinker and did not take drugs. As far as she knew, he had never experienced similar symptoms. Upon further questioning, she related that over the past several weeks, she and her husband had been having a serious marital argument (Greiner, 1964).

DISCUSSION OF CASE HISTORY #1

Initially, this patient received a diagnosis of acute schizophrenic reaction. But there is little evidence to support such a diagnosis. The sudden onset of *staggering incoherence* combined with clinical observations consistent with *visual hallucinations* and an *alternating level of consciousness* provide compelling evidence for an organic mental disorder. This is a classic picture of rapid onset brain syndrome. The dilated pupils suggest the possibility of drug intoxication. Unfortunately, the patient's vital signs were not reported; most likely, there would have been striking deviations in pulse, blood pressure, and temperature.

The man's wife finally reported that her husband had written a long letter the day he was brought into the hospital, addressed to his parents. The letter included the statement: "Whatever happens is not my wife's fault." She was instructed by the staff at the hospital to go home and search for signs of drugs or medications which might have been ingested. When she did so, she found a bottle in a wastepaper basket with a few remaining Sominex[R] tablets. Based on this new information, the clinical diagnosis was changed to acute scopolamine anticholinergic poisoning.

Within 24 hours the man had fully recovered.

Condition: organic mental disorder secondary to drug ingestion ("anticholinergic psychosis").

CASE HISTORY #2: THROWING IN THE TOWEL

A 33-year-old woman, without any history of significant mental or physical illness, was referred to a psychiatrist for her depression. She complained of losing interest in her work and in her friends. She also related how she had become obsessed with the possibility that her husband was being unfaithful—apparently, a concern not without some basis. This issue had led to many arguments that had become more intense over the past several months.

She complained of feeling trapped in her role as a housewife. She was drinking more but apparently not to excess. She denied any other drug use. There was no evidence of disturbances in memory or orientation. She appeared above average in intelligence. She denied any change in headache pattern. There were no deficits in speech, vision, or walking and no history of head injury or unexplained shifts in consciousness (Taylor, 1980).

DISCUSSION OF CASE HISTORY #2

The emergence of psychiatric symptoms for the first time at age 33 raises the suspicion of an organic mental disorder, but this was not confirmed by other findings.

With the patient's permission, supplementary information from a close friend was obtained. It substantiated the woman's account of her problem. No evidence for alcoholism or heavy drug use was found. Her suspicion regarding her husband was based in fact.

The woman entered psychotherapy and continued for 12 months. After painfully assessing her marital relationship (in the absence of her husband, who would not consider couple therapy), she decided to seek a divorce. Subsequently, she trained and was successful in securing a real estate license. Her depression disappeared.

After 2 years of living alone, she married a man whom she had dated for a year. She continued her career with considerable success.

Condition: Psychological reaction to marital problem.

CASE HISTORY #3: OUT OF CONTROL

Obviously out of control, a 25-year-old man was admitted to a hospital psychiatric service one week after completing Army summer camp. Within a few days of his return, he had begun to hear voices and to see things not visible to others. His wife described him as elated one moment and depressed the next. Finally, unable to resume normal work, he was taken by his family to an emergency psychiatric clinic.

When observed, he smiled inappropriately. He repeated himself over and over and was unable to provide any coherent information. At one point he had to be placed in seclusion for unmanageable behavior. Afterward, he was observed removing his clothes and assuming strange postures, some of which were clearly sexual in nature. When treated with chlorpromazine, he became much calmer and seemed generally improved.

Further questioning of the family established that his behavior was quite uncharacteristic. Although he was described as "fuzzy" on occasion, overall, his family portrayed him as reliable, stable, and without previous mental illness.

A thorough mental status examination demonstrated visual and auditory hallucinations with paranoid delusional thinking and an agitated, anxious demeanor. Periodically, the young man appeared confused, and was highly unpredictable (Penn, Racy, Lapham, Mandel, & Sandt, 1972).

DISCUSSION OF CASE HISTORY #3

The admission diagnosis was acute schizophrenic reaction, but this was changed to catatonic schizophrenia on the basis of the episodes of posturing, alternating with wild and violent behavior. On the third hospital day, the patient developed a fever. He became increasingly violent, despite electroconvulsive therapy. After steady deterioration in his condition, he died on the ninth hospital day, presumably of a severe, malignant, catatonic reaction.

At autopsy, however, evidence of a viral encephalitis was discovered. It was determined that there had been an outbreak of encephalitis in the summer camp area during the time the patient had been stationed there. Furthermore, it was learned that just prior to leaving camp, the patient had had a sudden episode of abdominal pain with body stiffness and a brief loss of consciousness. A medical evaluation at a nearby community hospital failed to turn up any basis for this attack. The recommendation that he have a follow-up assessment apparently was not pursued.

The *sudden onset* of uncharacteristic bizarre behavior with *no previous history,* in combination with clinical symptoms of *visual hallucinations* and *confusion,* strongly suggested organicity. *Fever* on the third hospital day (information the reader did not have) provided additional presumptive evidence of psychological masquerade.

Condition: Organic mental disorder secondary to viral encephalitis.

CASE HISTORY #4: IT COULD NEVER HAPPEN TO ME

A married man, age 34, a plumber by occupation, was seen for unexplained changes in his personality.

Throughout his initial interview, he sucked a red lollipop. In a slow monotone, he said that he felt anxious and physically ill. At one point he pulled out a bottle of methadone and started to drink it! He told how at age 29 he had first smoked heroin and then after the breakup of his first marriage, quickly progressed to I.V. use. He continued for the next five years (except for one year of self-imposed abstinence).

Later in the interview, he expressed his belief (incorrectly) that someone was "watering down" his methadone and selling it for a profit. He also recounted seeing bugs in his bed at night and hearing a stranger's voice. On mental status examination, given five objects to recall after five minutes, he could remember only three.

For the past 8 months, the man had suffered from a sore throat and had lost approximately 45 pounds. (Thomas & Szabadi, 1987).

DISCUSSION OF CASE HISTORY #4

There are several indicators of psychological masquerade. A man in his mid-thirties, with *no previous psychiatric history,* has an *unexplained* personality change. He has a *chronic sore throat associated with a 45 pound weight loss.* He is having *visual and auditory hallucinations and* on mental status examination can *remember only three of five objects.*

A medical evaluation turned up several important physical findings. White patches of discoloration were found in his throat. He was coughing up thick, green (obviously infected) sputum, and he had a widespread rash on his arms and chest.

Given his use of I.V. drugs (with its attendant risk of needle sharing), these physical findings were strongly suggestive of immunodeficiency. Laboratory testing confirmed a depressed white blood cell count and the presence of antibodies to the HIV virus. A CT scan demonstrated brain atrophy and dilated ventricles.

The patient was treated with an antifungal agent along with methadone, chlorpromazine and diazepam. At times he was confused, particularly at night. On one occasion he lost his way on the ward and could not find his own room.

He was transferred to a local infectious disease hospital but within a few days left against medical advice. At home he became increasingly disturbed, threatening his mother and resisting all medical help out of a belief that the visiting doctors were imposters. He had to be returned to the hospital against his will, where shortly thereafter he developed septicemia (blood infection). His condition rapidly deteriorated and he died. An autopsy showed that he had succumbed to pneumocystis carinii infection.

(As we will discuss later, a significant number of persons with AIDS have brain disease which can cause psychological masquerade.)

Condition: Organic mental disorder secondary to brain infection from HIV or an opportunistic infectious agent.

CASE HISTORY #5: HEAVY METAL

A 30-year-old woman became apathetic and socially withdrawn. She was unable to finish her housework. Even her personal appearance began to suffer. She would sit passively for hours in front of the television with her eyes closed. Her appetite was poor, and she had trouble sleeping. Often she would get up at night and pace the floor.

Eight years earlier, she had been treated in a psychiatric hospital for a "hysterical reaction." Her recovery from this episode was complete. She had had no further problems until the onset of her present symptoms. There was no history of substance abuse or serious medical illness. The only medication she was taking was an oral contraceptive.

Due to her current symptoms, she was readmitted to a psychiatric hospital. She was unkempt, drooling on herself, rigid in her posture with a fixed facial expression. She walked slowly, in a stooped fashion. Questions put to her were seldom answered. She avoided eye contact. Infrequently, she would mumble about being in hell and hearing the voice of the devil. Her memory, however, was intact and she was fully oriented. There was a mild tremor present in both hands. No other neurological abnormalities were present (Chung, Suseela, & Borge, 1986).

DISCUSSION OF CASE HISTORY #5

The woman was given a diagnosis of "functional psychosis," and treated (first with chlorpromazine and then with haloperidol 15 milligrams a day) without any improvement. In fact, on the fourth day, her symptoms became much more pronounced. She exhibited florid delusions and periodically screamed without provocation. At times it was necessary to restrain her. Her hand tremors became more severe until finally she could no longer hold her own cup and required assistance eating. A neurologist was consulted. He felt that she was having Parkinsonian side-effects from haloperidol. The medication was stopped.

When her condition still failed to improve, a full-scale neurological evaluation was undertaken which led to the true diagnosis. She was found to have a dramatic elevation in her urinary excretion of copper, and on split-lamp ophthalmoscopic examination, a Kaiser-Fleischer ring was seen in her cornea. She had Wilson's Disease, a genetic condition that leads to a destructive depositing of copper in body and brain tissue.

She was started on penicillamine (an agent which binds copper and facilitates its excretion from the body). She showed dramatic improvement in her psychiatric symptoms as well as her hand tremors and was discharged on a low copper diet along with her medication.

In this case the major clinical clues to psychological masquerade concern changes in body movement. The *rigid posture and stooped walking* in a 30-year-old woman, combined with *hand tremors,* are significant neurological findings that should not be overshadowed by more dramatic psychiatric symptoms. They signal organicity.

After four months, the woman had recovered sufficiently to allow her to return to work. One year later, her husband commented that she was in the best shape—emotionally and physically—she had been in since they were married.

Condition: Organic mental disorder secondary to Wilson's Disease.

REFERENCES

Chung, Y., Suseela, R., & Borge, G. (1986). Psychosis in Wilson's disease. *Psychosomatics, 27,* 65–66.

Greiner, T. (1964). A case of "psychosis" from drugs. *Texas State Journal of Medicine, 60,* 659–660.

Penn, H., Racy, J., Lapham, L., Mandel, M., & Sandt, J. (1972). Catatonic behavior, viral encephalopathy and death. *Archives of General Psychiatry, 27,* 758–761.

Taylor, R. (1980). Extracted from private clinical files.

Thomas, C., & Szabadi, E. (1987). Paranoid psychosis as the first presentation of a fulminating lethal case of AIDS. *British Journal of Psychiatry, 151,* 693–695.

Chapter 7

Four Masquerades

And after all, what is a lie? 'Tis but the truth in masquerade.
—Lord Byron

It is hoped, by this point, that the reader has accepted the proposition that organic disorders can capably masquerade as psychological problems. Fortunately, many of the disorders with the greatest propensity for masquerading are uncommon. Not so, however, with the four masqueraders we are about to consider: *brain tumors, epilepsy, endocrine disorders, and AIDS.*

In their most subtle guises, these masqueraders can fool even the most astute observer. Usually, however, they exhibit certain telltale clues of organic disease. Being on the lookout for these clues is the clinician's best guarantee against failing to recognize these masquerading conditions.

BRAIN TUMORS

Although brain tumors are not always malignant, they still can prove fatal. Roughly one out of five brain tumors are benign meningiomas—tumors of the outer coverings of the brain (Waggoner, 1967). If discovered early, such tumors usually can be removed, resulting in a complete cure. If the diagnosis is delayed, however, these tumors enlarge to a point at which treatment becomes mechanically impossible without gross destruction of surrounding brain tissue. In these tragic cases, the question of whether the tumor is malignant becomes immaterial. Early detection of brain tumors is essential.

Brain tumors are either primary or secondary. Primary tumors arise from brain tissue, whereas secondary tumors spread to the brain through a process of seeding from other parts of the body. The emergence of unexplained mental symptoms in persons with past histories of cancer suggests the possibility of a secondary brain tumor. This is especially true of breast and lung cancers.

Brain tumor symptoms arise primarily in one of two ways. First, depending on the exact location, local changes occur as a direct effect of the tumor. The expanding tumor may destroy brain tissue by invading, displacing, or compressing it within the closed space of the skull. In other instances nerve tracts in the oncoming path of the tumor are falsely stimulated. For example, if the tumor is located in the area of the brain related to visual perception, partial loss of vision or, more rarely, visual hallucinations may arise.

The second way a brain tumor produces symptoms relates to changes in the fluid pressure surrounding the brain. Tumor growth can cause significant increases in the intracranial pressure. Typically this leads to headache, vomiting, and blurred vision. Although these symptoms are considered classic manifestations of brain tumor, they do not always develop; and, even when they do, it may be extremely late. Of the three, headache occurs most consistently.

Approximately 60% of persons with tumors of the brain experience *headache* (Rushton & Rooke, 1962). In 20% of cases it is the *initial* manifestation (Gilroy & Meyer, 1973). The headache associated with brain tumor is highly variable in severity, but, with increased intracranial pressure, a recognizable pattern often emerges.

The headache is described as "pressure" or "throbbing." It is made worse by coughing, sneezing, straining, or exertion. Characteristically, the person finds that the pain is most severe upon awakening in the morning. Sometimes it even arouses the person from sleep. Typically, the headache will persist for several hours, gradually diminish, and disappear, only to recur the following day. Over time this symptom may last longer until it becomes persistent. The clinician should be alert to this ominous headache, which can be identified with a few elaborating questions concerning its quality, when it occurs, and what makes it worse. Other headache patterns, of course, should not be ignored, particularly when they are of *recent onset and are experienced by the person as unlike previous headaches.*

Another symptom highly suggestive of brain tumor is *seizure* (in the absence of an established history of epilepsy). Although seizures are not associated with brain tumor as frequently as are headaches, they are highly indicative of brain pathology. Seizures may be focal (localized) or generalized. If focal, the clinical picture reflects the area of tumor growth. Accordingly, the person may have abrupt episodes of involuntary movement, peculiar shifts in consciousness, or distortions in certain sensations. Generalized seizures, in contrast, produce a sudden loss of consciousness with total body collapse, followed by spastic jerking of the arms and legs. Either form of seizure should be considered indicative of organic disease. The reader may be surprised to find (as shown in several cases in this book) that seizures are sometimes misconstrued as being of minor consequence compared to the person's "psychological" symptomatology. This is a serious mistake.

Excessive drowsiness is yet another symptom seen with brain tumors. This symptom may lead to puzzling declines in a person's job performance or social life. Tolerance for alcohol and tranquilizing medication also markedly diminishes so that even small amounts produce drowsiness.

Finally, *elements of brain syndrome* are present in a high proportion of persons with brain tumor. In one study of 326 cases, 77% of the patients had some detectable cognitive deficit: 50% appeared confused; 39% were disoriented. Brain tumors with increased intracranial pressure are especially likely to produce brain syndrome.

Brain tumors located in areas primarily involved with motor movement or sensory perception stimulate changes easily recognized as neurological deficits; thus, with the possible exception of conversion reactions, these tumors are not often mistaken for psychological reactions. Tumors located in the frontal lobes are another matter.

Frontal Lobe Tumors

The frontal lobes encompass an extensive anterior area of the brain that is relatively "silent." This is not to say that nothing of neurological consequence is transacted in this area; it is after all, the part of the brain most involved in abstract thinking, judgment, and social propriety, as well as in the modulation of emotional expression. It is only silent in the sense that the deficits are not obvious neurological problems such as paralysis or sensory anesthesia. Technically, this silent area is the most forward portion of the front lobes, as opposed to a relatively smaller posterior area that includes the motor cortex. This is why, somewhat confusingly, the frontal area with which we are concerned is referred to as "prefrontal" (implying that it lies just anterior to the motor cortex).

During the clinical course of frontal lobe tumors, 70% of patients experience psychiatric symptoms. (Soniat, 1951) One researcher, reporting on 56 cases of frontal tumors, found that 46% of the patients initially received a psychiatric diagnosis. Mistaken diagnoses included depression (5 cases), presenile dementia (6 cases), schizophrenia (5 cases), anxiety state (2 cases), and inadequate personality (1 case). (Kanakaratnam & Direkze, 1976).

Two contrasting psychiatric syndromes have been described in frontal tumors. The more common of the two is characterized by depression, apathy, indifference, emotional flatness, reduced spontaneity, and sometimes diminished intellectual ability. Understandably, such cases can be mistaken for psychological depression.

> At retirement age, a government clerk was referred to a local emergency room by his family physician with a note stating that the man should be admitted to the psychiatric service for treatment of severe depression.
>
> A more extensive history revealed that for more than 3 years the man had suffered from excessive drowsiness, unusual for him prior to that time. For the past 2 months, he had had severe headaches and had undergone brief periods of memory loss and confusion. Apparently, these symptoms had played a major role in his recent failure to obtain a job promotion.
>
> In the emergency room, he was uncooperative. He was described as depressed and easily irritated. A cursory neurological examination failed to show any abnormalities. But based on his history of deteriorating cognitive performance, a brain scan was requested, which identified a "space-occupying lesion."
>
> At surgery a right frontal lobe tumor (astrocytoma) was removed. The man recovered without complications and, subsequently, was described by his wife as his old self. (Carlson, 1977)

The recent onset of severe headaches in combination with sudden shifts in consciousness and a history of increased drowsiness, provided the basis for a strong suspicion of organicity.

The second clinical picture seen in frontal lobe tumors is somewhat the opposite. The person becomes euphoric and light-hearted. Often this devil-may-care, don't-give-a-damn attitude leads to antisocial or outright criminal behavior. Social and sexual inhibitions disappear, and the person's personal hygiene may suffer. This pattern resembles that found in manic reactions. In some instances the euphoria evolves into a silly, childish manner with intellectual decline.

The following case illustrates the manic features sometimes prominent in cases of frontal lobe tumor.

> After a brief observation period during which he was agitated, talking rapidly in nonstop fashion and compulsively naming objects, a 29-year-old veteran was admitted to a V.A. hospital. When asked what his problem was, he replied: "Nothing sir, just ignorance; just gross ignorance around here." His response to a question about his occupation was: "I was a carpenter, like Jesus." He

alternated between statements suggestive of a grandiose view of himself and thoughts of persecution. He was fully oriented and had no difficulty with memory. His judgment, however, was poor.

His medical records showed a 6-year history of seizures thought to be related to drinking. These seizures usually began with a peculiar feeling of strangeness, followed by loss of consciousness, collapse to the floor, and jerking of his arms and legs. Despite these seizures, he had been sent overseas during World War II and during an 11-month period reportedly had suffered no further episodes. Upon discharge he received a 50% service-connected disability for "neurosis." The seizures subsequently resumed.

Three months prior to his admission, the man was seen in a psychiatric outpatient clinic for intractable anxiety. Gradually, his condition progressed to severe restlessness, agitated elation and flights of ideas. After taking a leave of absence from his job, at home he became openly hostile and belligerent. He went without sleep and soon became unmanageable, necessitating hospitalization.

Neurological studies—including an EEG and pneumoencephalogram—led to a tentative diagnosis of frontal lobe tumor, confirmed at surgery when a "parasagittal meningioma" was removed from the right frontoparietal area. One month later, the man's mental condition appeared entirely normal. (Oppler, 1950)

This was a difficult case. The clues to its organic origins were limited. The key was the history of seizures for which no explanation had been provided other than that they might be related to drinking. This man had a six-year history of seizures, which in all likelihood reflected the slow growth of a meningioma. Meningiomas are the most common form of frontal lobe tumor.

The relatively silent nature of the frontal area makes it imperative that the clinician be familiar with those few neurological deficits that do arise. A brief recap of certain anatomical aspects of the frontal lobes is in order. Along the medial aspect of the frontal lobes, on either side, is situated a micturition center, crucial to voluntary control of the bladder. This area is a favorite site for meningiomas; thus it is not unusual at some point for the person to lose bladder control. *Mental symptoms associated with incontinence should always be considered organic.*

The major nerves and brain tracks involved in smell and sight maintain a close anatomical juxtaposition to the underside of the frontal lobes. For this reason, frontal tumors may produce changes in vision and, more rarely, smell. Connections also exist between the frontal lobes and parts of the brain involved in walking. When these connections are disrupted, deficits appear similar to those seen in Parkinson's disease: shortening of steps and a progressive loss of balance.

Although the precise mechanism is unknown, frontal lobe tumors sometimes trigger catatonic-like episodes.

At age 22 the woman began to have peculiar attacks during which she was unable to move or speak. Periodically, while eating, she would suddenly go into a daze, dropping the eating utensils from her hands. In addition she complained of vague sensations in her head as well as attacks of sleepiness. Her condition was thought to be psychological. She was treated briefly by a hypnotist without any change. Within a short time she began to hear strange voices muttering obscenities. Eventually, she notified the police that she was being victimized.

Six months later, preoccupied with bodily sensations and constantly hallucinating, she was admitted to a psychiatric hospital. Her report read: "hallucinated in all senses, worried by visions of wild animals and indecent sexual activities."

On the unit she accused doctors and nurses of playing with her brain. She felt that her eyes were "being made to work in Morse code." At times she was frankly catatonic. Her diagnosis was schizophrenia.

Twelve years later, still in the hospital, she was claiming to be a lieutenant in the Army as well as a psychologist at Cambridge, Horatio Bottomley's sweetheart, and heiress to the British throne.

After 17 years she had become impulsively violent, and all her somatic complaints were being interpreted by the staff as psychotic productions.

So accustomed were her doctors to regarding her utterances as manifestations of a sick mind that when she complained of failing sight they noted: "Still wildly deluded—she believes she cannot see her own image in the mirror."

After 26 years of institutionalization, this woman received a neurological examination that showed the nerves conducting visual impulses from her eyes had completely deteriorated (optic atrophy). Even then (unbelievably!) she was still presumed to be schizophrenic. Only after she began to have generalized seizures was she transferred to a research hospital, where studies showed a large intracranial mass identified at surgery as a frontal lobe meningioma. It proved to be inoperable. The woman never regained consciousness; she died 2 days later. (Hunter, Blackwood, & Bull, 1968)

This case extended over 43 years! For virtually this entire period—despite such clues as sudden shifts in consciousness with muscle weakness, visual deterioration, attacks of drowsiness, and generalized seizures—the diagnosis of schizophrenia was doggedly maintained. This case convincingly illustrates the slow-growth pattern of meningiomas. It also shows how a false diagnosis can blind us to obvious signs of organicity.

Limbic System Tumors

The limbic system consists of a group of interrelated brain structures primarily concerned with individual and species survival. Primitive human drives, with their attendant emotions, arise in this ancient brain system (MacLean, 1964). When tumors develop in the limbic brain, manifestations are often dramatic behavioral–emotional responses, such as fear or rage.

Since the limbic system is highly compact anatomically, even extremely small tumors cause significant emotional changes. Eventually, if these tumors remain undetected, eating, sleeping, drinking, and sexual behavior may also become disturbed.

A study of 18 patients with limbic tumors showed that in all cases an initial psychiatric diagnosis had mistakenly been given: schizophrenia (10 cases), depression (4 cases), severe neurosis (3 cases) and mania (1 case) (Malamud, 1967).

The following is an example of a limbic tumor mimicking a problem of psychological sexual dysfunction.

> A 36-year-old married man with sexual impotence was referred for psychiatric treatment. Married for 13 years, he had two children. His work history was exemplary, and he did not appear to be under any unusual stress.
>
> Sixteen months prior to his referral for treatment, the man began to experience gradual decline in sexual interest. Within 5 months, he was unable to obtain an erection at any time. He also had attacks of anxiety, "feelings of dread" that persisted for 5 to 6 seconds and then disappeared. These episodes increased in intensity until eventually they became full-fledged panic attacks. Sometimes an attack would be preceded by the "compulsion to stare" and by the feeling that everyone else was going through a similar experience. The man's wife noticed that during these attacks her husband underwent a sudden blanching of his face and stopped talking.
>
> After a complete medical evaluation, a limbic brain tumor was diagnosed and surgically removed. The man's recovery was rapid. He had no further episodes of panic, and his sexual interest returned. (Johnson, 1965)

The temporal lobes have the highest incidence of tumors directly connected to the limbic system. If the tumor happens to involve the posterior aspect of the left temporal lobe, fluent aphasia is likely to result. The reader will recall from our previous discussion that this condition can be extremely misleading because it is easily mistaken for psychotic speech.

Many temporal lobe tumors stimulate seizure activity, thereby producing a clinical picture identical to temporal lobe epilepsy (complex partial seizures), a disorder that we will take up in detail in the next section.

A 53-year-old man with no previous psychiatric history began to have "spells" during which he heard strange musical sounds. He would then become overwhelmingly depressed. The depression and the musical sounds would disappear after a short while, but the spells recurred with increasing frequency. Eventually, the man was committed to a state hospital with the diagnosis of involutional depression.

Over the next 3 months, he became lethargic and developed a pronounced weakness in his left arm and leg. Eventually, he slipped into a coma, and died. At autopsy, a large tumor of the right temporal lobe was discovered. (Malamud, 1967)

This man had no previous psychiatric history. His "involutional depression" was highly atypical in that he experienced it in short-lived episodes, and the auditory hallucinations were not consistent with a depressed mood. These findings argued against a psychological depressive reaction.

Before proceeding to our next masquerader, perhaps a brief summary of what we have said about brain tumors would be worthwhile. Table 7.1 gives a concise overview. Brain tumors are not rare conditions, and any brain tumor can give rise to psychological symptoms, although this is more typically the case in tumors of the frontal, limbic, and temporal areas. I have emphasized the importance of headache, seizures, drowsiness, and brain syndrome as clues to brain tumors. Slow-growing, benign meningiomas represent approximately 20% of all brain tumors, and their favorite place of occurrence is the frontal area, where they produce two distinctive patterns of mental and emotional changes: apathetic depression and antisocial mania. Encroachment on the "nonsilent" areas of the frontal lobes may provide important clues such as urinary incontinence, abnormal movement, deficits in vision and smell, disordered speech, and catatonic-like behavior. Finally, limbic system tumors can give rise to powerful emotional and behavioral changes.

EPILEPSY

A seizure is an electrical discharge within the brain giving rise to movement, feelings, or thoughts unrelated to the external situation. In other words, seizures are a kind of short-circuiting of the brain. They result from a variety of causes, including infection, tumors, hypertension, hemorrhage, trauma, and drug intoxication and withdrawal. in the majority of cases, however, no precise explanation can be established. Such cases are referred to as idiopathic epilepsy.

TABLE 7.1 Brain Tumors

Suggestive Findings

General
  Headache
  Seizures
  Drowsiness
  Brain syndrome

Frontal Lobes
  Two characteristic clinical patterns:
    Apathetic-depressive
    Antisocial-manic
  Loss of bladder control
  Shortening of walking steps
  Deficits in vision and smell
  Catatonic reactions

Limbic System
  Strong emotional discharges
  Disturbances in instinctual behavior: eating, drinking, sex, aggression
  "On-off" shifts in consciousness or perception
  Aphasia (left temporal lobe)

The outward manifestations of seizures depend on the site of involvement. The most common type is grand mal epilepsy. Such seizures are global brain discharges involving virtually the entire cerebral cortex, including, most dramatically, the motor cortex. The seizure typically begins with the person feeling somewhat strange. He may cry out and then lose consciousness and, if standing, fall to the floor. The muscles of the body undergo a brief but sustained spasm followed by a wave of short jerking movements in the arms and legs that usually subside after a few minutes. The person is unconscious for this entire sequence and retains no memory for what has transpired. The only exception would be memory for the first few seconds of the seizure. The person may experience one of a variety of strange senations (known as an aura) just at the outset of the seizure. Since the individual is fully aware during this brief prelude, this is the last thing remembered.

In addition to the dramatic jerking movements, during a grand mal seizure the person may also drool, make biting movements, and lose bladder or bowel control. As the seizure subsides, the person appears flushed. Over a period of several minutes, consciousness is regained, but usually with some residual confusion. During this twilight period, strange behavior stemming from the person's confusion may occur. Sometimes this phase is more drawn out, resulting in a sustained period of erratic behavior and incoherent speech suggestive of schizophrenia. Suspiciousness and unprovoked aggression may also emerge, reflecting the person's uncertainty about the situation.

Although grand mal epilepsy can be mistaken for psychological reactions (particularly when the person is observed during the period immediately following the seizure), this potential is considerably greater in complex partial seizures.

Complex partial seizure is the official neurological designation for what is more popularly known as temporal lobe epilepsy or psychomotor seizure. This term has been selected to emphasize the intertwined cognitive and behavioral (complex) aspects of this type of seizure, while at the same time indicating its circumscribed nature (partial) as contrasted to grand mal epilepsy. Anatomically, these seizures arise in the limbic system with its temporal connections. Table 7.2 summarizes the factors suggestive of this disorder that will be discussed here in more detail.

The area having the greatest propensity for complex partial seizures are the temporal lobes, a sizeable extension of the limbic system. The temporal lobes play a pivotal role in perceptual integration. It is here that various kinds of sensory information are synthesized and interpreted. Highly unusual and distorted perceptions arise in temporal lobe epilepsy during the aura. Abruptly, without explanation, the person experiences strange perceptions. Although a wide range of perceptual changes are possible, typically, in any given individual the same subjective sensation is repeated each time.

The person may feel as though he is in a dream. A sense of familiarity may engulf him so that a situation experienced for the first time seems as though it is the recurrence of a past situation (deja vu); or the opposite

TABLE 7.2 Complex Partial Seizures

Suggestive Findings

Temporal Lobe Epilepsy
  Unprovoked, episodic behavioral changes
  Trance-like appearance
  On-off shifts in consciousness or perception
  Stereotypical movements of the face and neck

Episodic Dyscontrol
  Unprovoked spells of violence associated with an altered state of consciousness
  Precipitation by alcohol or minor tranquilizers

perception may occur, so that the person suddenly has a sense of strange-ness despite familiar surroundings. Powerful emotions may erupt; feelings such as fear, loneliness, sadness, or anger. Sometimes visual changes dominate the aura. Objects may seem far away and small; or, the opposite, close at hand and gigantic. Sounds may become extremely muted or very loud. Strange voices or musical sounds are sometimes heard. The person's body may feel distorted. A sense of abdominal distress may grip the person. Foul smells are particularly common, often described as the smell of "rot-ting eggs" or "burning rubber." The aura or first phase of a temporal lobe seizure usually lasts only a matter of seconds and is immediately followed by a second phase.

The second phase also persists for only a matter of seconds. It is charac-terized by the person's loss of awareness. Often, this is manifest by a blank stare. If the person has been talking, his speech may be abruptly inter-rupted, although in some cases the person will continue to verbalize inco-herent, repetitive sounds making for a confusing clinical picture.

The third stage is the longest. It may persist for several minutes and, in exceptional cases, for hours. The primary manifestation is automaton-like behavior. Particularly common are movements of the neck and face: lip-smacking, teeth-grinding, chewing, tongue-sucking, and jerky, turning mo-tions of the neck from side to side. These movements are the most defini-tive clinical signs of temporal lobe epilepsy, but they can be quite subtle. In rare cases highly complicated sequences of behavior lasting for hours have transpired: activities such as driving an automobile or performing surgery!

The fourth and final stage is a gradual transition over several minutes. The automatic activity recedes, and consciousness returns. The person feels groggy and, other than the initial aura, has little memory for what has transpired.

Clinicians, more often than not, are presented with a history of strange "spells" that they are not able to observe first hand. It is this history of on—off behavior, uncharacteristic of the person and inappropriate to the situa-tion, which must capture the clinician's attention if he or she is to recognize a seizure disorder.

A single man in his early twenties was admitted for the *thirtieth time* to a psychiatric service. These admissions had occurred over a 5-year period and always involved the same bizarre, hyperactive, frenzied behavior. The man was well known to the local police as well as the hospital staff.

The patient was started on what had become a routine treatment plan for his "schizophrenic episodes," beginning with 100 mg. of chlorpromazine (IM) and seclusion in a side room until the medication could take effect. On this particular admission, due to a shortage of beds, the patient was sent to a different ward, where he was evaluated by a physician who had never before been involved.

The patient was "muttering, grunting, groaning, or humming" as he rolled and crawled on the floor. At times he made masturbatory gestures and pelvic thrusting movements of a sexual nature. He was also noted to have strange expressions on his face, sucking, blowing, and grinning in peculiar fashion. He scratched and scraped the walls, muttering over and over again: "Hare Krishna, Hare Krishna, Hare Krishna . . ." But within 3 hours, this strange behavior had disappeared.

As though awakening from a turbulent sleep, the patient rubbed his eyes and calmly asked for a cigarette. The psychiatrist judged him at this time to have no disturbance in thought, mood, or speech. There was only the faintest recollection of what had transpired over the past several hours. The patient was removed from seclusion and spent five days on the psychiatric service without showing any further symptoms.

A thorough review of his hospital records revealed (in 12 volumes) a variety of diagnoses, including: acute schizophrenia, chronic undifferentiated schizophrenia, psychotic reaction, obsessive–compulsive personality and, on his most recent previous admission, "hypomania in the context of chronic schizoaffective illness." The pattern of events leading up to each hospitalization was virtually identical. He would suddenly experience auditory hallucinations after which he would run wildly down the street in the nude.

Despite this exhaustive rereview, the patient was again discharged without detection of his real problem. Ten days later, however, he was readmitted for similar symptoms and (based on the observations recorded during the previous admission) was moved to a long-term unit for careful observation. In a relatively short period, five additional episodes had taken place. They were judged to be identical reruns of each other. All attacks were ushered in by a period of withdrawn behavior, during which the patient expressed feelings of hopelessness and became increasingly less coherent. Invariably, the full-blown picture of bizarre behavior and strange movements appeared within a matter of minutes or hours.

Despite several attempts, no seizure pattern was found on the patient's EEG; nevertheless, based on clinical observations, a diagnosis of complex partial seizure was made. Three subsequent seizures were quickly terminated with a rapidly acting antiepileptic agent (diazepam). During a 6-month follow-up period, the patient was successfully controlled on an antiepileptic medication (acetazolamide). (Adebimpe, 1977)

This case well illustrates several key aspects of complex partial seizures. The dramatic contrast in the patient during the episode and afterwards— the on–off effect—is an extremely important finding and should always alert the clinician to the possibility of seizures. Acute psychiatric disruptions seldom have the "rerun" quality of seizures. In addition, they rarely ever resolve in the course of a few hours. In the foregoing case, the man went from being wildly psychotic to completely normal within a 3-hour period. Even drug-related psychiatric disturbances usually require a longer period for resolution as the drug clears the system.

The reader should not assume that all cases of complex partial seizures have four clearly definable stages. Wide variations in clinical presentation occur. Virtually any of the characteristic symptoms can become the most prominent aspect of an individual's seizures. Given the myriad of connections between the temporal lobes and other parts of the limbic system, unusual clinical presentations are to be expected. Take the following case:

> A woman called the police after (for the second time in a single week) her neighbor's husband removed his clothes in his back yard and exposed his genitalia to her. The man was taken into custody. An investigation turned up additional information. A police report had been filed four months earlier after the man was found standing motionless by the roadside, naked from the waist down. Furthermore, under more intensive questioning, his wife related that approximately one year earlier without any explanation he removed all his clothes in front of his children. She said he appeared confused.
>
> A psychiatrist evaluated the man and diagnosed him as a case of exhibitionism.
>
> Further neurological evaluation was performed, however, when it was found that at 17 years of age the man had been knocked unconscious for several minutes by a falling tree. An EEG showed a wave and spike pattern over the left temporal area. A revised diagnosis of temporal lobe epilepsy was made. He was started on Dilantin®, and after almost two years of follow-up, had had no further episodes of exhibitionism. (Hooshmand, & Brawley, 1959)

The most important clinical clue to the epileptic nature of these episodes was the confused, trance-like state that came over the patient. An additional important fact was the history of having lost consciousness for several minutes following a severe blow to the head. Head trauma sometimes leads to scarring of brain tissue and years later causes seizures.

Another form of epilepsy (presumably originating in the limbic system) presents as rage attacks. These episodes of violence last from a few seconds to hours. Often, the attack is completely unprovoked; in other instances, a minor provocation will precipitate a vicious assault. The use of alcohol and minor tranquilizers increases the frequency of these violent seizures. Sometimes, the individual will show an extremely low tolerance for such drugs, so that even minimal usage brings on an attack.

This condition has been termed *episodic dyscontrol* (Bach-y-Rita, Lion, Climent, & Ervin, 1971). Persons suffering from it often have a history of childhood hyperactivity, arrest records for violence-related crimes, extensive traffic violations, and automobile accidents. The attacks are commonly preceded by a trance-like state or aura, which may consist of visual hallucinations, body numbness, or a heightened awareness of sounds. Once the episode is terminated, the person may complain of drowsiness or a headache and has no memory for what has transpired. The strongest evidence for the epileptic nature of episodic dyscontrol is derived from treatment responses to antiepileptic medication.

In one study of 22 persons with episodic dyscontrol, after two months of treatment with an antiepileptic medication (Dilantin®), 19 of the patients had shown at least a 75% reduction in the frequency and severity of their attacks (Maletzky, 1973). This is a particularly impressive finding given that these persons had previously received other forms of therapy without beneficial results. (On the other hand, this was not a controlled study.)

Repeated instances of unprovoked, violent outbursts, especially when associated with shifts in consciousness and intensified by alcohol or tranquilizers, suggest the possibility of episodic dyscontrol.

> A 23-year-old, unemployed mechanic beat his wife with a metal candlestick, causing multiple lacerations and loss of consciousness. Afterward, the wife recalled how he initially "went into a blank stare" prior to attacking her.
>
> The same man fatally shot his best friend. Abruptly, for no reason, he grabbed the man's hunting rifle and shot him. This happened shortly after the two of them had finished drinking a couple of cans of beer. He was jailed but released on bond. Shortly afterwards, he hurled his daughter out of the window of a moving automobile. His explanation was that she had "talked back."
>
> This man had a history of childhood truancy and hyperactivity. He quit school in his early teens and had been jailed on numerous occasions for assault and drunken driving. He was evaluated by a psychiatrist and determined to have episodic dyscontrol. (Maletzky, 1973)

Consider a second example.

> He referred himself for treatment, complaining that he was anxious. He was having intrusive thoughts of self-destruction, and most disturbing of all, episodes of violent behavior. The man was 25 years old and unmarried. He had completed several years of college where he studied electronics. Currently, he was employed as an electrical technician, a job which he described as stressful.
>
> There was no additional history of psychiatric disorder. He denied using drugs.
>
> Several months earlier while at work he started having intrusive thoughts; vivid suicidal fantasies in which he would visualize himself with his throat slit, bleeding to death. About the same time, another recurring thought began to bother him. As he drove home from work, he would cross a train track at

which point a visual image would flash into his mind of himself being hit and horribly crushed by an oncoming train.

He denied actual hallucinations or delusions. But his ability to concentrate had suffered considerably; and, at work he was having frequent staring spells.

Several weeks after first seeking psychological help, he was traveling in a car with members of his family. When his brother nonchalantly addressed a comment to him, without any warning, he became terribly upset, shouting and threatening the others in the car. In a rage he broke his own glasses. Before the car came to a complete stop, he jumped out, slamming the door on his grandmother's ankle. Other similar unprovoked episodes followed.

When questioned, the patient said he was unaware while these incidents were actually happening. He did describe, however, a "funny feeling" or "buzzing in his head" a few minutes before they occurred. Afterwards, he felt drained physically and emotionally. There had been no instances of loss of consciousness or incontinence.

On examination he was alert, fully coherent and oriented. An EEG was ordered. During hyperventilation (a procedure performed to bring out EEG abnormalities) it showed bursts of 6/second spike and wave complexes. Sleep recordings showed 6 and 12 rhythmical sharp waves in the mid-temporal areas.

Given the clinical history and these EEG abnormalities, treatment was started with carbamazepine (Tegretol®), an antiepileptic medication. Ten months later the EEG pattern was normal, and the patient had had no further outbursts or staring spells. He was continued on medication indefinitely. (Stone, McDaniel, Hughes, & Herman, 1986)

Despite such cases, the reader should recognize that the relationship between violence and epilepsy is not well established. This is a controversial topic among neurobehavioral specialists. Violence and epilepsy need to be kept in perspective: The vast majority of persons who are violent are not violent because of seizures; conversely, most persons who suffer from epilepsy are not violent.

ENDOCRINE DISORDERS

Hormones exert powerful emotional and behavioral effects. The slightest imbalances can result in dramatic psychological and cognitive changes as well as alterations in physical appearance (Smith, Barish, Correa, & Williams, 1972). Such changes are seen with numerous endocrine disorders. In this section, we will focus on three that occur with some frequency. We will review *hypoglycemia, hyperthyroidism, and hypothyroidism*. These conditions provide the reader with examples of the tremendous masquerading potential of endocrine disorders generally.

Hypoglycemia (Low Blood Sugar)

The simple sugar, glucose, is the essential nutrient of the nervous system. Whereas other parts of the body readily utilize alternative sources of energy, the nervous system relies almost exclusively on glucose, requiring a constant supply for normal functioning. This statement about the essential reliance of the nervous system on sugar may strike the reader as difficult to reconcile with all the nutritional warnings about the dangers of excessive sugar consumption. It is true that the body can be overwhelmed by large loads of glucose, thus setting into play a series of disrupting hormonal changes. Also, pure sugar provides calories without any other nutritional value, so called naked calories, so that overreliance on sugar leads to nutritional deficiencies. In order for the nervous system to be assured of an optimal supply of energy, a variety of food substances can be consumed in the diet and later converted into glucose as the demand arises. Nevertheless, glucose, itself, is essential; the brain must have a stable supply. Situations leading to wide fluctuations in blood glucose levels create neurological havoc.

Hypoglycemia is not a specific disease; rather, it is a physiological condition—a syndrome—that can result from a variety of causes. If the organs responsible for the absorption of glucose from ingested food fail to perform, hypoglycemia results. Similarly, if the pancreas—the endocrine gland that manufactures and releases insulin, the major regulator of glucose—becomes overproductive, low blood sugar ensues. If the liver in its role as a storage reservoir for glucose in the form of glycogen fails to function properly, hypoglycemia again is the consequence. Hypoglycemia can also be a man-made problem, as when excessive amounts of insulin are taken by persons with diabetes mellitus. This results from errors in dosage or from a change in factors affecting the amount of insulin required. Insulin overdoses are probably the most common precipitants of hypoglycemia. Diabetics are at high risk.

Regardless of the specific cause, hypoglycemia evokes a powerful emergency response from the sympathetic nervous system. This automatic discharge is targeted at counteracting hypoglycemia. Outwardly it is expressed as perspiration, tremulousness, increased heart rate and blood pressure, dilation of the pupils, and a subjective sense of feeling ill, usually with nausea and anxiety. If hypoglycemia persists, after a time the initial sympathetic reaction subsides, giving way to more flagrant mental symptoms resulting from the brain's dwingling energy supply. At this juncture the person may show an extremely diverse group of symptoms, including confusion, bizarre behavior, irrational fear, delusions, hallucinations, and, in the most serious cases, coma. These manifestations of hypoglycemia have misled even the finest clinicians. If detected, however, the emergency treatment is simple and immediately effective, but first, the clinician must correctly identify the problem.

Some of the most dramatic recovery stories from hospital emergency rooms relate to cases of hypoglycemia. The person may have been found wandering on the street; perhaps brought in by the police. In the absence of any medical history, the clinician is confronted with an incoherent individual who appears quite crazy. Preparation is made to admit the person to a psychiatric unit, blood is drawn for a series of routine laboratory tests; then, if the individual is lucky, the physician injects an intravenous solution of glucose. This is a common procedure adopted by physicians who recognize the tremendous masquerading potential of hypoglycemia. Within minutes—sometimes even seconds—this psychotic person becomes sane. Calmly and coherently, the person inquires as to what is going on, since his memory for what has transpired is usually defective. No trace of bizarre behavior remains. The person may relate, as is so often the case, that he is a diabetic and recently has had trouble regulating his daily dose of insulin. Obviously, given what has transpired, he took too much.

Hypoglycemia also can result from tumors that secrete insulin-like substances. Consequently, the person develops an excess of insulin-hormone activity and resulting low blood sugar. A review of 91 cases of insulin-producing tumors showed that 40% initially had been misdiagnosed, half of them being mistaken for functional psychiatric problems (Laurent, Debry, & Floquet, 1971).

A young man in his early twenties with a history of excellent health underwent a personality change. He complained of weakness, especially in the morning upon awakening. On one occasion he mysteriously fainted while shaving.

Over a 3-month period, he had episodes of confusion. Although after these bouts of confusion, he appeared like his old self, he could never recall what had happened. Gradually, he became withdrawn and negativistic in his relationships with his family.

Finally, he was taken to a hospital where he was thought to be having a schizophrenic break. Despite treatment, however, he became more unresponsive and withdrawn. One morning he was found in a coma. Upon receiving a 50% glucose solution intravenously, within a matter of minutes he fully recovered. His blood sugar level was found to be one-third of normal.

A complete medical workup turned up a large, previously undetected mass in his lower posterior abdomen which at surgery was diagnosed as a retroperitoneal fibroma. The tumor had been secreting an insulin-like substance, accounting for the episodes of hypoglycemia.

Eighteen months later, the man reported no further problems. He had returned to full-time employment. (Silvis & Simon, 1956)

I do not wish to leave the reader with the idea that hypoglycemia always creates dramatic or psychotic behavioral changes. To the contrary, this condition is capable of producing much more subtle alterations such as irritability and nervousness. In this form hypoglycemia is considerably more difficult to recognize as a psychological masquerade.

No precise cause can be identified for "reactive hypoglycemia." Although it is not as common as the popular press suggests, it does occur. It is presumed that persons with this problem are physiologically predisposed to periods of low blood sugar. It is thought that the body overreacts to sugar (particularly after the ingestion of food with a high sugar content) with an excessive production of insulin that in turn, causes a precipitous drop in blood sugar. Symptoms from reactive hypoglycemia typically include anxiety, irritability, and a sense of not feeling well. In more severe cases, cognitive deficits occur. The person may find it difficult to concentrate and think through simple problems. He may become suspicious and develop mental confusion and memory gaps.

The next case is an unusual history. I have included it not as a representative example of reactive hypoglycemia but rather as an illustration of the far-ranging clinical presentations associated with this baffling disorder.

As she was nearing her home on a return trip from a nearby neighboring town, a woman was stopped in her automobile by the local police. They were investigating a hit-and-run accident that had resulted in the death of a cyclist earlier in the evening. Upon being questioned, the woman recalled passing the scene of the accident; but, seeing that help had arrived, she decided not to stop.

She was a social worker by training, the wife of a practicing family physician, well respected in her community, a "citizen of excellent character." She fully cooperated with the police, even submitting to two breath analyzer tests for alcohol (negative results). The police then escorted her home, where they continued to question her about the accident. After more than an hour of extensive interrogation, the questioners were unable to detect any knowledge on her part of the occurrence of the accident, although the woman readily admitted that she had likely been in the area at the time the fatality happened. Within a few days, however, incriminating evidence surfaced when damage to her car was linked to the scene of the crime.

This woman had no official history of psychiatric disease, but her close friends and family described what they considered "uncharacteristic behavior" over the preceding three years. During these periods, she had difficulty completing her thoughts and was easily irritated. She would become irrationally suspicious, angry, and even threatening but then, usually within a short period, would seem her normal self. She apparently had no recall for these stormy altercations, at least she never mentioned them.

On occasion she complained of nausea and appeared tremulous, suggesting to those who knew her well a bit of a hangover. Even her complaints of exhaustion and depression and her attacks of breaking out into a cold sweat were considered the product of drinking too much. Although the woman, herself, admitted to the regular use of alcohol "as a sedative" before going to bed, she firmly denied drinking to excess.

During the days immediately preceding the accident, she had been under considerable stress, preoccupied to the extent of failing to eat properly. In fact, on the day of the accident, she had not eaten anything. When she left for the neighboring town, her family noticed that she was not quite herself, but no one felt that she was incapable of driving.

Due to the inconsistencies in this case, an extensive medical examination was requested. A 5-hour glucose tolerance test demonstrated a profound re-bound hypoglycemia (30 mg%) four hours after the ingestion of a standard glucose meal. This finding led to a diagnosis of reactive hypoglycemia. The court accepted a plea of guilty, imposed a nominal fine, and disqualifed the woman from driving because of her hypoglycemic disorder. (Bovill, 1973)

Two factors in this case should be emphasized. The regular use of alcohol and extended periods without food commonly aggravate reactive hypoglycemia. In the foregoing case, the woman had gone most of the day without eating, thereby predisposing her to hypoglycemia. (Somewhat paradoxically, symptoms also tend to occur several hours after a heavy intake of sugar, as illustrated in the special glucose tolerance test performed on this woman. This is the result of excessive release of insulin.) Also, despite her protestations, there was evidence that this woman drank alcohol to excess.

Hypothyroidism (Myxedema)

The hormone regulating a person's metabolic rate is produced by the thyroid gland. Too much produces a revving up of the body; with too little, body functions are slowed.

The thyroid gland is situated in the midline of the neck at the level of the Adam's apple. It comprises two lobes, one on either side of the windpipe, connected by a narrow bridge of tissue. Unless abnormally enlarged, the gland cannot be seen; in certain disorders, it may be observed as a prominent bulge in the neck.

Hypothyroidism is a state of thyroid deficiency. It can result from different diseases and also, ironically, as the aftermath of treatment for an overactive thyroid gland. This treatment is difficult to administer precisely. Too much of the thyroid gland may be destroyed, leading years later to hypothyroidism.

Regardless of the specific cause, hypothyroidism characteristically has a gradual onset. Symptoms may appear one after the other, making it difficult to surmise that they all stem from the same cause. There is an overall slowing of physiological functioning. It is as through the body's "pacemaker" has been turned down, so that the processes of life go on at a much slower pace. The heart rate is slowed; the blood pressure depressed. The gut becomes sluggish, causing constipation. Because less energy is expended, the person gains weight despite maintaining his or her usual food intake. The body temperature is lowered, leading to complaints of feeling cold when others are comfortable or even overly warm. The person may have the subjective sense of being slowed down. Fatigue is common.

Women develop hypothyroidism five time as often as men. Frequently, they complain of changes in their menstrual period, particularly excessively flow.

Despite the numerous somatic changes seen with hypothyroidism, psychological symptoms are often the most prominent findings. Typically, the person feels blue. The ability to concentrate and solve simple problems may be compromised. At this stage, hypothyroidism can be mistaken for a depressive reaction.

> A 48-year-old housewife noticed that her energy was gone. She found herself easily fatigued, listless, and irritable. In looking for a likely explanation, she blamed her symptoms on menopause, even though her menstrual periods remained unchanged. Finally, she went to her physician, who told her that she was depressed and started her on a tricyclic antidepressant medication. Her symptoms persisted.
>
> Eventually, she sought out a second physician, who upon hearing her story and observing certain physical changes—paleness in her skin color and a puffiness about her face—decided to evaluate her thyroid gland. The laboratory results confirmed hypothyroidism. She was started on thyroid hormone, and her symptoms disappeared. (Martin, 1979)

As hypothyroidism deepens, a person's physical appearance undergoes significant changes. The skin becomes dry and thickened, taking on a creamy hue, especially noticeable in the face. The hair grows brittle and dry and begins to shed. Puffiness develops in the face, especially prominent in the eyelids. The eyebrows thin and the outermost portion may even fall out. The person's voice deepens, becoming husky and raspy, making his or her speech difficult to understand.

Psychological changes show a similar intensification and can reach psychotic proportions ("myxedema madness"). Paranoid delusions are often prominent and can lead to "retaliatory" violence. The psychotic symptoms sometimes mask a decline in intelligence, which if treated early enough is usually reversible.

> Following a rageful attack during which furniture was destroyed and family members threatened, a middle-aged man was forcefully admitted to a mental hospital.
>
> Eight years earlier, this previously healthy and highly productive gentleman, an academic administrator, complained of fatigue and a peculiar tingling sensation in his arms. A medical examination failed to identify any problem.
>
> Over the next several years, the patient underwent a number of changes. He became sluggish of movement and his intellectual ability declined. He grew suspicious of people and eventually exhibited angry tantrums, during which he smashed things about the house and on occasion, beat his wife. His outward appearance slowly changed. His skin grew pale, dry, and excessively wrinkled; he gained weight, and his hair started to fall out.
>
> When admitted to the hospital, the man was noted to have blatant paranoid delusions and to speak in a deep, husky voice. (Olivarius & Roder, 1970)

Found to have severe hypothyroidism, he was started on treatment with replacement thyroid hormone. Ten weeks later he was discharged. At that time he was described as mentally normal. Within 6 months his weight and appearance had also returned to normal. He successfully resumed his work in academic administration. (Given the long delay in diagnosis and treatment, this case had an unusually satisfying outcome.)

Unfortunately, the tests routinely used for thyroid screening purposes fail to pick up marginal cases of thyroid dysfunction, known as "occult" hypothyroidism. In a study of 15 consecutive depressive patients (all women), unresponsive to medication, researches discovered that despite having normal levels of the two main thyroid hormones (T3 and T4), one-third were in fact hypothyroid. (This was established by measuring the metabolic rate and TSH, a hormone not routinely used as a thyroid screen.) These women fell into a pattern of being overweight, sluggish, bothered by obsessional ruminations and slowed thinking. Their depressions responded favorably to treatment with thyroid hormone (Gewirtz et al., 1988).

As evidenced in the following case history, depression is not the only symptom associated with "occult" hypothyroidism.

> A hearing-impaired 65-year-old woman became convinced that her food was being poisoned by strangers living in her attic. Her family described her as increasingly agitated, often unable to sleep. She had been observed responding to what appeared to be auditory and visual hallucinations. Treatment with thiothixene (20 milligrams a day) proved ineffective.
>
> After being hospitalized, she was disoriented, confused, and very sad. When she spoke it was usually about losses she had sustained in her life.

Standard thyroid tests, including T3, T4, and free thyroxine, were within normal limits. Her TSH level, however, was markedly elevated, indicative of hypothyroidism. It was also determined that four years earlier, thyroid hormone had been prescribed for the patient. She had taken it for only a short time and then stopped for no apparent reason.

Within one week, treatment with thyroxine produced dramatic changes. The woman's mood improved and her delusional beliefs began to resolve. Her discharge diagnosis was organic brain syndrome secondary to hypothyroidism. (Haggerty, Evans, & Prange, 1986)

One final point. Lithium preparations (widely prescribed for affective disorders) can induce hypothyroidism, usually after several years. In one study of 116 lithium-treated patients, thyroid evaluation turned up hypothyroidism in roughly 8% of cases. The average duration of lithium therapy was 3.4 years (Yassa, Saunders, & Camille, 1988). Any person taking lithium who begins to experience mental dullness, apathy, depression, sensitivity to cold, or unexplained weight gain should be checked for hypothyroidism. It's an iatrogenic condition easily confused with psychological depression.

Hyperthyroidism (Thyrotoxicosis or Graves' Disease)

Hyperthyroidism is roughly the flip-side of hypothyroidism. The body's metabolic rate is increased. The pacemaker seems to be stuck in an "up" position, so that excessive caloric energy is continuously consumed. It is as though the person is being readied for a stress or struggle that never materializes. The boiler room is working overtime.

As with hypothyroidism, hyperthyroidism develops much more often in women than in men. It appears most commonly at puberty and in middle life and, of special interest to the clinician, it frequently is preceded by a severe emotional stress.

The physical symptoms can be quite prominent, but, as with other masqueraders, such symptoms are often neglected due to the overshadowing psychological changes. The individual sweats excessively and is overly sensitive to heat. The heart rate, blood pressure, and temperature are often elevated. A fine tremor in the hands is typical and the person's eyes sometimes become prominent, even bulging. The skin is flushed and *warm*, in contrast to the cold and clammy skin condition associated with acute anxiety. Often, despite a voracious appetite, there is a history of weight loss. Insomnia may be a problem. The same for heart palpitations and shortness of breath. Women undergo changes in their menstrual pattern; some may even stop having a monthly menstrual flow.

The most characteristic mental and emotional expressions of hyperthyroidism are anxiety, irritability, and a kind of emotional fragility, characterized by crying or laughing without provocation. Despite the overall appearance of tension and nervousness, the person often describes an uncomfortable sense of *energized fatigue*. The simultaneous occurrence of restless anxiety and exhaustion should suggest the possibility of hyperthyroidism. The cognitive changes vary from mild distractibility to paranoid delusions and symptoms of brain syndrome.

In cases that persist for an extended period, the clinical picture may shift to one of depression and apathy. It is as though the prolonged hypermetabolic state eventually exhausts the body's reserves. This somewhat paradoxical presentation of hyperthyroidism has been described frequently in elderly persons, and is often misdiagnosed as depression or dementia.

Occasionally, hyperthyroidism is mistaken for a manic reaction. Although the hyperthyroid person may become expansive and grandiose, this is almost always *without* the element of euphoria typical of mania.

> For no apparent reason, the wife of a resident physician began to feel extremely anxious. She had difficulty sleeping and at times was tremulous and given to heavy perspiration. She felt exhausted much of the time.
>
> Eventually, she brought herself to discuss these symptoms with her husband, who interpreted them as signs of the stress of being a resident's wife. He started her on a minor tranquilizer for her "anxiety."
>
> But her symptoms did not improve. In fact, the woman became more agitated, anxious, and obsessed with the thought that she was probably losing her mind.
>
> Finally, almost as a self-fulfilling prophecy, she was admitted to a psychiatric hospital. No significant "emotional conflicts" were identified. Instead, she was found to have an elevated heart rate and an unexplained weight loss. Laboratory studies established that she was suffering from hyperthyroidism. She was treated with radioactive iodine, after which her "anxiety" disappeared. (Martin, 1979)

A recent study of 13 untreated cases of hyperthyroidism makes clear that this condition is a spectrum disease, capable of diverse psychiatric presentations. The researchers found nine patients with major depression; eight generalized anxiety disorder; four, panic attacks; and three, hypomania. Even more confusing, 7 of the patients met the criteria for *both* major depression and generalized anxiety disorder (Trzepacz, McCue, Klein, Levey, & Greenhouse, 1988). The psychological manifestations seen in hyperthyroidism are not restricted to anxiety and hypomania. The apathetic depression described in elderly persons also appears with almost equal frequency among younger persons. Being sensitive to a mixed clinical picture of anxiety and depression in combination with the characteristic somatic changes is the key to recognizing hyperthyroid masquerade.

TABLE 7.3 Endocrine Disorders

Suggestive Findings

Hypoglycemia
Episodes of sweating, nervousness, and nausea
Unusual behavior after long periods without food, relieved by eating
Unusual behavior a few hours after heavy intake of sugar
Unusual behavior in a person with diabetes mellitus

Hypothyroidism
Depression with weight gain, sensitivity to cold, and characteristic physical changes
Previous history of treatment for hyperthyroidism
Intellectual decline with characteristic physical changes

Hyperthyroidism
Unexplained anxiety or manic behavior with *warm*, flushed skin
Energized fatigue
In older population, unexplained apathetic depression with intellectual decline

Of further interest, this study reported no psychotic symptoms. While there is no doubt that hyperthyroidism can manifest as functional psychosis—both schizophreniform and affective—this occurs in a minority of cases, but it is important to recognize because when psychosis results from an overactive thyroid gland, thyroid ablation (either surgical or medical) is curative.

Hyperthyroidism has been associated with other psychiatric presentations, including anorexia nervosa, periodic catatonia, and rapid cycling bipolar disorder (Byerky, Black, & Grosser, 1983; Gjessing, 1974).

Taken together, endocrine disorders (especially thyroid) accounted, in one major study, for over 20% of psychological masquerades. Hormones have powerful effects on the brain as well as the body. When they are out of balance, mental and emotional dysfunction can be suspected (Hall, Popkin, DeVaul, Faillace, Stickney, 1978). Table 7.3 provides a concise summary of the major symptoms of Endocrine Disorders discussed above.

AIDS

AIDS (Acquired Immunodeficiency Syndrome) is a life-threatening disease caused by human immunodeficiency virus (HIV) infection, resulting in a breakdown of the body's immunity. When immunosuppression reaches a critical point, the person becomes susceptible to a host of opportunistic infections as well as cancers such as Kaposi's sarcoma.

HIV infection is spread through intimate sexual contact and blood exchanges, such as occurs when common needles are used by individuals who are shooting drugs. In this country gay men, IV drug users, prostitutes and other persons who have intimate sexual contact with people in these groups are at highest risk for contracting AIDS. No one, however, is invulnerable. It is not who you are but rather what you do that determines risk for AIDS.

Coming to grips with having AIDS (and for others, living with the ever-present threat), can elicit painful psychological reactions, experienced as anxiety, panic, depression, or grief. Additionally, persons infected with the HIV virus are vulnerable to organic mental disorder.

It is not clear what percentage of persons exposed to HIV will develop AIDS, but for those who do come down with the disease, likely, it will happen several years after they have been infected. The initial symptoms include some or all of the following:

- night sweats
- unexplained weight loss and fatigue
- fever
- unusual infections, particularly of the mouth
- purplish skin blotches
- persistent diarrhea

In 60% of AIDS cases, *pneumocystis carinii* pneumonia is the initial presenting problem. Usually, there is a gradual onset of malaise followed by a cough, low-grade fever, and generalized chest pain.

Initially, it was believed that HIV exclusively infected T-cell helper/inducer lymphocytes, thereby immobilizing the body's immunological defenses against a host of potential pathogens. It is now clear that HIV infection is not limited to the immune system. Brain cells are also susceptible. In addition, many of the opportunistic organisms that attack the body when it is in a state of immunosuppression can also cause brain infections. Add to these potential causes of organic mental disorder, invasion of the brain by tumors (particularly lymphomas) and it becomes clear why a majority of persons with AIDS exhibit neuropsychiatric symptoms (Perry & Jacobson, 1986; Fenton, 1987).

In one study, 29 patients at high risk for AIDS initially presented with cognitive or behavioral symptoms (Bradford & Price, 1987). Six of them had no other clinical manifestations. All of the patients had some degree of cognitive impairment. In the early stages this was limited to poor concentration, mild memory problems, and mental slowing. Emotional changes were prominent early features, leading to the diagnosis in the three cases. Over a third had notable personality changes. With time more severe manifestations of brain syndrome appeared. Seven patients experienced paranoid psychosis.

Depression commonly antedates the onset of AIDS, but brain syndrome is the most common organic mental presentation. Sometimes it results from infections of the coverings of the brain—meningitis—involving agents such as cryptococus or herpes simplex virus; or, from infections of the brain itself with syphilis, toxoplasmosis, or tuberculosis. But the most common etiology of brain syndrome is the "subacute encephalitis" that presumably is caused by HIV.

This condition has been called "AIDS dementia complex" (ADC). The clinical picture involves a mix of cognitive, motor, and affective disturbances. Studies have shown that 35–50% of AIDS patients with neurologic complications have ADC (Broder, 1987). When cognitive deficits rapidly emerge, delirium results, with confusion, disorientation, delusional thinking, and hallucinations. The more characteristic pattern is an insidious onset over many months.

It often starts with difficulty concentrating. The process of thinking, itself, may be sluggish (bradyphrenia). Gradually, problem solving is compromised. Routine matters become confusing. Memory begins to fail. The person's emotional responses are blunted, until finally there is little reaction to events that earlier would have elicited strong emotion. The person's energy level drops. Apathy and withdrawal from social involvement are predictable. Sexual interest shows a notable decline and may disappear altogether. At this point the person's condition can be mistaken for depression. In fact, depression may be a part of this clinical picture, but it is occurring as one aspect of a serious disruption in cognitive functioning.

Along with these changes, the person usually loses his coordination. Walking becomes slow and unstable; handling objects such as utensils in the kitchen is increasingly problematic. Involuntary movements, such as tremors, may appear. Often, there is considerable weight loss and the person becomes frail.

In some patients this progressive decline will be intermittently punctuated by psychotic symptoms which mimic schizophreniform, paranoid, or manic reactions.

Given the guarded prognosis for AIDS patients, psychological reactions would be expected. It is unclear how often this is a response to the stress of coping with a life-threatening disease as opposed to being a sign of brain pathology. Certainly, severe depression, mania, or paranoid reactions in persons at high risk for AIDS should suggest the possibility of an unrecognized HIV infection or secondary complication.

> After three months of progressively becoming more and more depressed, a homosexual man in his mid-thirties was admitted for psychiatric treatment. There was no previous psychiatric history.
>
> For some time he had complained of fatigue and a loss of strength in his arms and legs. He had lost a noticeable amount of weight. His previous medical history included hepatitis and, one month before his admission, a yeast infection of his throat and esophagus.
>
> His physical examination showed a low-grade fever and swollen lymph glands. He looked emaciated. There were no obvious neurological deficits.
>
> During his interview, the patient looked directly ahead with a blank, wide-eyed stare. His speech was slow, as were his body movements. Other than a reflex-like smile that infrequently crossed his face, he was without animation or spontaneity. He did not speak unless questioned and then would give only one- or two-word replies. His recent memory seemed intact, and there were no hallucinations or delusions.
>
> On three occasions the patient's EEF failed to record any abnormalities. A CT scan, however, showed diffuse cortical atrophy and enlarged ventricles, indicative of significant brain pathology.
>
> The patient remained in the hospital for seven weeks, eventually becoming mute and profoundly confused and disoriented. He was finally discharged to a convalescent hospital where (after four months) he died of pneumonia secondary to AIDS. (Hoffman, 1984)

Consider a second example of AIDS masquerading as a psychiatric disorder.

> Abruptly, out of the blue, a young man in his early 20s became grandiose and pressured. He went without sleep. His mind seemed to go nonstop. He wouldn't finish one thought before going off on something else. He seemed completely different from his old self. Now he was easily irritated, preoccupied with sex, and constantly concocting elaborate and completely unrealistic schemes. He spent money he didn't have and eventually began to hear voices that weren't present.
>
> His condition escalated, and finally psychiatric hospitalization was required. Clinical evaluation confirmed his "hypomanic" symptoms. Otherwise, he was fully alert, oriented, and capable of abstract problem solving. His physical examination and a battery of laboratory studies, including thyroid tests, were normal, as was his CT scan.
>
> There was no previous psychiatric history and no family history of affective disorder. He admitted to drug use but said it had been restricted to the occasional recreational use of cocaine and marijuana. He was bisexual.
>
> There was rapid and dramatic improvement in response to treatment with a neuroleptic drug. After the addition of lithium carbonate, however, the patient

had a serious reaction with fever, sweating, and muscular rigidity, consistent with the clinical picture of neuroleptic malignant syndrome, a relatively rare but life-threatening adverse reaction to neuroleptic medication. All medication was stopped.

Within a few days, the patient became agitated and psychotic again. Various treatments were employed, including amobarbital, lorazepam, and two courses of electroconvulsive therapy (ECT), without beneficial results. The patient remained in the hospital.

Four months later tests showed evidence of immunosuppression (T4/T8 cell ratio inversion) which had not been present previously. Within two weeks, he came down with *pneumocystis carinii* pneumonia and later developed purplish skin blotches (Kaposi's sarcoma). The pneumonia was successfully treated, but the patient still was unable to leave the hospital. Three months later he remained physically debilitated, depressed, and cognitively compromised. (Gabel, Barnard, Norko, & O'Connell, 1986)

A final point to keep in mind with respect to AIDS relates to adverse effects to medication. AIDS patients are exquisitely sensitive to psychotropic medications. (As in the above case, there have been a large number of reported cases of neuroleptic malignant syndrome in AIDS patients.) Overdosage is a common problem in the psychopharmacological management of psychosis, depression, or anxiety. In addition, because of the various infections and cancers that may complicate these cases, patients are at considerable risk for requiring treatment with neurotoxic agents, providing yet another basis for organic mental disorder. This includes pentamidine (Pentam 300) in *pneumocystis carinii*, amphotericin B in cryptococcus and oral candidiasis, isoniazid (INH) in tuberculosis alpha-interferon in Kaposi's sarcoma, and azidothymidine (AZT) and zidovudine (Retrovir) against HIV infection.

Given the projected increase in the number of persons with AIDS, psychological masquerade secondary to HIV will become common.

The capacity for masquerading is by no means limited to the conditions we have considered in this chapter; but, I trust that the discussion of brain tumors, epilepsy, endocrine disorders, and AIDS—in addition to providing the reader with specific information about these four masqueraders—will serve to broaden the reader's overall clinical perspective on the problem of psychological masquerade.

REFERENCES

Adebimpe, V. (1971). Complex partial seizures simulating schizophrenia. *Journal of the American Medical Association, 237,* 1339–1341.

Bach-y-rita, G., Lion, J., Climent, C., & Ervin, F. (1971). Episodic dyscontrol: a study of 130 violent patients. *American Journal of Psychiatry, 127*, 49–54.

Bovill, D. (1973). A case of functional hypoglycemia—a medico-legal problem. *British Journal of Psychiatry, 123*, 353–358.

Bradford, N., & Price, R. (1987). The acquired immunodeficiency syndrome demential complex as the presenting or sole manifestation of human immunodeficiency virus infection. *Archives of Neurology, 44*, 65–69.

Broder, S. (1987). *AIDS, Modern Concepts and Therapeutic Challenges.* New York: Marcel Dekker.

Byerley, B., Black, D., & Grosser, B. (1983). Anorexia nervosa with hyperthyroidism: case report. *Journal of Clinical Psychiatry, 44*, 308–309.

Carlson, B. (1977). Frontal lobe lesions masquerading as psychiatric disturbances. *Canadian Psychiatric Association Journal, 22*, 315–318.

Fenton, T. (1987). AIDS-related psychiatric disorder. *British Journal of Psychiatry, 151*, 579–588.

Gabel, R., Barnard, N., Norko, M., & O'Connell, R. (1986). AIDS presenting as mania. *Comprehensive Psychiatry, 27*, 251–254.

Gewirtz, G., Malaspina, D., Hatterer, J., Feureisen, S., Klein, D., & Gorman, J. (1988). Occult thyroid dysfunction in patients with refractory depression. *American Journal of Psychiatry, 145*, 1012–1014.

Gilroy, J., & Meyer, J. (1973). *Medical Neurology* (3rd Ed.). New York: Macmillan Publishing Co.

Gjessing, L. (1974). A review of periodic catatonia. In Kline, N. (Ed.), *Factors in Depression*, (227–249). New York: Raven.

Haggerty, J., Evans, D., & Prange, A. (1986) Organic brain syndrome associated with marginal hypothyroidism. *American Journal of Psychiatry, 143*, 785–786.

Hall, R., Popkin, M., Devaul, R., Faillace, L., & Stickney, S. (1978). Physical illness presenting as psychiatric illness. *Archives of General Psychiatry, 35*, 1315–1320.

Hoffman, R. (1984). Neuropsychiatric complications of AIDS. *Psychosomatics, 25*, 393–400.

Hooshmand, H., & Brawley, B. (1959). Temporal lobe seizures and exhibitionism. *Neurology, 19*, 1119–1124.

Hunter, R., Blackwood, W., & Bull, J. (1968). Three cases of frontal meningiomas presenting psychiatrically. *British Medical Journal, 3*, 9–16.

Johnson, J. (1965). Sexual impotence and the limbic system. *British Journal of Psychiatry, III*, 300–303.

Kanakaratnam, G., & Direkze, M. (1976). Aspects of primary tumors of the frontal lobe. *British Journal of Clinical Practice, 30*, 220–221.

Laurent, J., Debry, G., & Floguet, J. (1971). *Hypoglycemic Tumors.* Amsterdam: Excerpta Medica.

MacLean, P. (1964). Man and his animal brains. *Modern Medicine, 3*, 95–106.

Malamud, N. (1967). Psychiatric disorder with intracranial tumors of limbic system. *Archives of Neurology, 17*, 113–123.

Maletzky, B. (1973). The episodic dyscontrol syndrome. *Diseases of the Nervous System, 34*, 178–185.

Martin, J. (1979). Physical diseases manifesting as psychiatric disorders. In G. Usden & J. Lewis (Eds.) *Psychiatry in General Medical Practice.* (337–351).

Oivarius, B., & Roder, E. (1970). Reversible psychosis and dementia in myxedema. *Acta Psychiatrica Scandinavia, 46*, 1–13.

Oppler, W. (1950). Manic psychosis in a case of parasagittal meningioma. *Archives of Neurology and Psychiatry, 64,* 417–430.

Perry, S., & Jacobson, P. (1986). Neuropsychiatric manifestations of AIDS—spectrum disorders. *Hospital and Community Psychiatry, 37,* 135–142.

Rushton, J., & Rooke, E. (1962). Brain tumor headache. *Headache, 2,* 147.

Silvis, R., & Simon, D. (1956). Marked hypoglycemia associated with nonpancreatic tumors. *New England Journal of Medicine, 254,* 14–17.

Smith, C., Barish, J., Correa, J., & Williams, R. (1972). Psychiatric disturbances in endocrinologic disease. *Psychosomatic Medicine, 34,* 69–86.

Soniat, T. (1951). Psychiatric symptoms associated with intracranial neoplasm. *American Journal of Psychiatry, 106,* 19–22.

Stone, J., McDaniel, K., Hughes, J., & Herman, B. (1986). Episodic dyscontrol and paroxysmal EEG abnormalities: successful treatment with carbamazepine. *Biological Psychiatry, 21,* 208–212.

Trzepacz, P., McCue, M., Klein, I., Levey, G., & Greenhouse, J. (1988). A psychiatric and neuropsychological study of patients with untreated Graves' disease. *General Hospital Psychiatry, 10,* 49–55.

Waggoner, R. (1967). Brain syndromes associated with intracranial neoplasm. In A. Freedman & H. Kaplan (eds.), *Comprehensive Textbook of Psychiatry,* (786–791). Baltimore: The Williams & Wilkins Co.

Yassa, R., Saunders, C., & Camille, Y., (1988). Lithium-induced thyroid disorders: a prevalence study. *Journal of Clinical Psychiatry, 49,* 14–16.

Chapter 8

Drug-Induced Organic Mental Disorders

There are some remedies worse than the disease. —Publilius Syrus

Drugs and medications cause organic mental disorders; furthermore, they frequently do so without being recognized—thus the need for a special chapter devoted to drug-induced psychological masquerade.

Under the designation *drugs* we will consider a variety of chemical substances in three categories: psychiatric prescription medications, general prescription medications, and street drugs. Our discussion will not be comprehensive, but rather a selective consideration of those drugs with a special propensity for causing mental and emotional changes. From the outset, however, a key point should be emphasized: *With respect to psychological masquerade, any drug is suspect.*

Even when assured that the information will be held in strict confidence, people underreport their use of drugs. A study of 225 persons entering a community mental health program found that 13% were covertly using hard drugs (opiates, cocaine, and amphetamines); that is, they had not shared this practice with their therapists (Hall, Popkin, Stickney, & Gardner, 1978).

Failure to disclose drug use is not restricted to illicit drugs and is not always the result of deception. Sometimes a person taking a substance simply does not think of it as a drug. This is particularly common with over-the-counter medications, which, unfortunately, can produce serious side effects. Certain medications may not be mentioned because the individual separates physical health concerns from mental and emotional problems. Medicine taken regularly for high blood pressure, for example, may go unidentified because the person sees no relevance to his or her "psychological" problem for which help is being sought.

In other instances a person may actually be unaware that a particular substance is being taken into the body. For example, parents may have no idea that their child is intoxicated with lead as a result of eating lead-based paint off the apartment walls. Similarly, an employee may unknowingly absorb an industrial or agricultural toxin as he goes about his work. A person may report the use of one drug, such as marijuana, unaware that it has been laced with strychnine or PCP.

In addition to the pervasive and often hidden nature of drugs, clinicians should be sensitive to the untoward effects drugs sometimes exert on one another. One drug may increase or decrease the effect of another drug, or when taken simultaneously, the two may produce an entirely different reaction. As more and more potent drugs are produced, the risk of hazardous drug–drug interactions increases. In mental health care, this has emerged as a significant complication due to a tendency toward multiple-drug treatment.

PSYCHIATRIC PRESCRIPTION MEDICATIONS

Most psychiatric medications can have adverse side effects. Improvement in the target symptom should not keep the clinician from observing new symptoms caused by the medication itself. Untoward effects often occur simultaneously with the desired action.

Neuroleptics

Neuroleptics (also called antipsychotics or major tranquilizers) are routinely prescribed for the management of psychotic behavior. Table 8.1 contains a selective list. A number of side effects are encountered, some dose related, but not all. Certain individuals simply have an extreme sensitivity to these drugs and react adversely to even low doses.

Parkinsonian reactions occur with considerable regularity, particularly in young persons treated with high-potency neuroleptics. These side effects may abruptly emerge, often within a few days of the initiation of treatment. When full-blown, they can be extremely frightening. In dystonic reactions, the person's neck haltingly twists to one side, as though being pulled by an invisible force. The torso may twist to one side. Speech may be garbled due to muscle incoordination and involuntary protrusion of the tongue.

Because this strange complex of symptoms typically occurs while the patient is being treated for psychotic behavior, the clinician runs the risk of

TABLE 8.1 Neuroleptics (Selected list)

High potency		Low potency	
haloperidol	(Haldol®)	thioridazine	(Mellaril®)
fluphenazine	(Prolixin®)	mesoridazine	(Serentil®)
thiothixene	(Navane®)	chlorpromazine	(Thorazine®)
molindone	(Moban®)		
loxapine	(Loxitane®)		

mistaking this reaction for "bizarre behavior" or "posturing," a symptom seen in catatonic schizophrenia. Because of the dramatic overlay, parkinsonian effects can be misconstrued as hysterical behavior. Sometimes, a single dose is all it takes to produce a reaction. This is an important point because neuroleptics commonly are used in emergency rooms for the treatment of nausea and vomiting. Acute parkinsonian symptoms may develop later after the patient has gone home. (Patients should be warned that this is a possibility.) When the patient returns for help, the connection with the medication may be overlooked and this bizzare reaction erroneously labeled a psychiatric problem, as occurred in the following unfortunate case.

> Having bitten her tongue several times, an agitated mentally retarded teenager was seen in an emergency room. After her tongue was sutured, she was sent back to the nursing home where she lived, whereupon she promptly bit her tongue almost completely through, requiring 50% surgical removal. An ER physician interpreted her tongue-biting as a psychological reaction to her dislike of the nursing home!
>
> Several days later, a psychiatric consultation was requested. A review of the patient's record showed the following. Four days earlier she had had fever with vomiting for which she received prochlorperazine, 10 mg initially and then 5 mg three times a day until she was seen in the emergency room. The night before, she had cried and complained of how painful her tongue was as it protruded from her mouth. Although it was obvious that she was biting it, the staff (not understanding that this was caused by the medication she was taking) did nothing. (Meyers, 1988)

Neuroleptics can cause brain syndrome, particularly in older persons. The risk of this complication is greatly increased when these medications are given in combination with an antidepressant or antiparkinsonian agent, as this raises the likelihood of anticholinergic toxicity.

A 23-year-old man had been treated for several years by a local mental health agency for impulsive and psychotic behavior.

One evening he was brought involuntarily to a hospital, violently agitated and disoriented, showing signs of visual hallucinations. His pupils were widely dilated, his pulse 120 beats per minute, and his temperature elevated.

Recently, the young man had been taking multiple medications, including haloperidol, thioridazine, and an antiparkinsonian agent.

After emergency treatment with physostigmine (an anticholinergic "antidote"), the patient's psychotic behavior resolved, and his vital signs returned to normal. (Granacher, & Baldessarini, 1975)

This problem could have been mistaken for the reemergence of psychosis. Fortunately, it was correctly diagnosed as an anticholinergic psychosis.

Anticholinergic side-effects merit extra comment. These troublesome side-effects are commonly experienced by patients receiving tricyclic antidepressants or low-potency neuroleptics such as thioridazine and chlorpromazine. Additionally, there is a class of drugs specifically referred to as "anticholinergics." They play a prominent role in psychiatry because they act as "antidotes" to the parkinsonian symptoms associated with high potency neuroleptics.

These medications are additive in their anticholinergic effect. Anticholinergic side-effects are particularly problematic for older persons, often causing confusion and frank psychosis, even when employed in relatively small amounts. (Anticholinergics are also found in over-the-counter medications, although in recent years they have increasingly been replaced by other medications. Diphenhydramine, however, continues to be widely available in sleeping preparations and in anti-allergy and motion sickness medications.)

Reports of the intoxicating properties of anticholinergics date back to ancient times. Found in certain plants scattered throughout the world, these substances, with their delirium-inducing powers, were mentioned in Chinese and Sanskrit writings; and Homer, in the *Iliad* and the *Odyssey*, portrayed their potent effects.

Anticholinergic effects are portrayed in the following rhyme:

> Mad as a hatter,
> Blind as a stone;
> Red as a lobster,
> Dry as a bone.

(Back in the 19th century, the art of hat-making required exposure to highly neurotoxic mercurial compounds; consequently, going "mad" became a recognized occupational hazard associated with hat-making.)

Less florid cases of anticholinergic toxicity show mild disorientation, apathy and drowsiness. In their most dramatic expression, mental changes take the form of a delirious psychosis, with frightening visual hallucinations. The pupils become widely dilated and remain unaffected by bright lights which normally cause the pupil to constrict. In addition, the small muscle controlling the thickness of the lens becomes paralyzed, preventing appropriate accommodation and leading to blurred vision.

Frequently, the person's skin will flush, especially about the face, probably as a result of the dilation of small blood vessels. With the elevation in temperature seen in these cases, one would expect to find increased sweating. Not so. Perspiration is characteristically absent, despite fever. The combination of mental confusion, widely dilated pupils, elevated temperature, and *decreased* sweating strongly suggests anticholinergic drug intoxication.

> A 17-year-old man was forcibly brought to an emergency room. Disoriented to time and place, he also exhibited delusional thinking, agitation, and hallucinations, both visual and auditory. At times the patient's agitation erupted into frank assaultive behavior. His pulse was 120, and he was noted to have widely dilated pupils. His skin was flushed and warm; but despite a rectal temperature of 105°F, he showed no signs of perspiration.
> The following morning the man was completely lucid. He reported that he had purchased Asthmador® pipe tobacco from a local shop, returned home; and, rather than smoke it, he had used the tobacco to brew a tea-like drink. He "freaked out" after drinking one cup of this unusual brew, hallucinating strange things crawling on his body. (Shader & Greenblatt 1971)

Designed for asthmatics, Asthmador® is a special pipe tobacco containing anticholinergic medication which allegedly reduces the irritating effects of pipe smoking. This man's unorthodox and ill-advised use of Asthmador® resulted in a classic case of anticholinergic psychosis.

High potency neuroleptics (particularly in large doses) can produce a bizarre, rigid posturing resembling catatonic schizophrenia and often mistakenly treated with higher doses. The person assumes frozen postures for extended periods, usually without speaking or acknowledging others. Even if the person is able to speak, the complaint of this strange experience is likely to be misinterpreted as "crazy."

> Five years earlier, a 44-year-old woman was hospitalized for severe obsessive–compulsive symptoms. She received more than 60 electroconvulsive treatments with "moderate improvement."
> Gradually, over the next several years, her obsessive–compulsive behavior returned, until finally she was rehospitalized and treated with Haldol®, 20 mg daily.

After discharge, she continued the medication, but her obsessive–compulsive symptoms returned and along with them, a robot-like appearance. She stood motionless, drooling on herself. Eventually she lost control of her bowel and bladder, necessitating rehospitalization.

When interviewed, she was rigid and motionless, staring ahead with her mouth open. She had difficulty speaking and could not, on her own, initiate body movement. From time to time, she assumed strange postures.(Gelenberg & Mandel, 1977)

The medication was stopped, and she was given amantadine (Symmetrel®), an antiparkinsonian drug. Within three days the woman was speaking in her normal voice; and after one week, she no longer showed rigidity, posturing, or difficulty initiating movement. Although she continued to have obsessive–compulsive symptoms, she required no maintenance medications.

Akathisia—a relentless, internal restlessness—is a frequent and bothersome consequence of neuroleptics, leading many individuals to stop their medication. This excruciating restlessness often causes endless pacing, one of the few activities that provides relief. This symptom can be mistaken for anxiety and interpreted as an indication of the need for additional medication, thus setting into place a vicious cycle.

Akathisia likely explains many episodes of "loss of control" in persons taking neuroleptics. Regrettably, restraints and locked side-rooms often are employed inappropriately, simply because akathisia is not recognized. You can imagine the frustration and anger felt by the person who is the target of this kind of clinical mistake.

An on-call physician was paged by the night staff, requesting a "stat" order for antipsychotic medication. An earlier admission, an eighteen-year-old high school senior with numerous psychiatric hospitalizations for schizophrenia, was "about to blow." He was described as showing "imminent assaultive potential."

When the physician reached the unit, he found the patient pacing back and forth in front of the nurses' station, shouting that it had been a mistake to sign himself into the hospital. He said he couldn't stand "being cooped up" and "needed out right away."

It was determined that one week earlier he had received a neuroleptic (fluphenazine decanoate, 1cc intramuscularly) and had been started simultaneously on an antiparkinsonian drug, three times daily. On the day of his hospital admission he had received another injection of the neuroleptic, but had missed taking the parkinsonian antidote. Even though the patient showed no obvious physical signs of parkinsonism (such as rigidity or tremor) the examining physician surmised that he was experiencing akathisia as a drug reaction to fluphenazine.

Within half an hour of receiving the antiparkinsonian medication, the patient stopped pacing the floor and appeared much calmer. He went to bed and within a short time fell asleep. (Siris, 1985)

Akathisia is easily overlooked. It should always come to mind when patients receiving neuroleptics become anxious, fidgety, or agitated.

The lower potency neuroleptics have different problems. Breast enlargement (gynecomastia)—sometimes with lactation—is not infrequent. When this occurs along with failure to menstruate (another side effect seen with these medications), the uninformed patient may assume erroneously that she is pregnant. Men also experience their share of bothersome symptoms, such as difficulty achieving an erection or ejaculating. These problems have been extensively reported with thioridazine (Mellaril).

When taken for extended periods, neuroleptics carry a significant risk for tardive dyskinesia, especially in older persons. Tardive dyskinesia is a condition of purposeless, jerking, twitching movements, usually most severe in the muscles of the tongue, face, and extremeties. A person with moderate to severe tardive dyskinesia may also manifest lip smacking, blowing of the cheeks, tongue protrusion and grinding movements of the chin and jaws. Writhing movements in the arms and legs or around the torso of the body also occur, though less commonly. At a minimum tardive dyskinesia causes embarrassing disfigurement. In rarer cases, it becomes disabling and even life-threatening.

With continued use of neuroleptics, eventually, tardive dyskinesia becomes irreversible. For this reason it is essential that the clinician recognize its cardinal signs so that, if at all possible, treatment can be discontinued. It is important to remember that tardive dyskinesia, oddly enough, is improved with higher doses of neuroleptic; thus, the causative agent, temporarily at least, gives symptomatic improvement. So, if tardive dyskinesia has developed, it will most likely be observed when a patient has stopped his medication or has recently reduced the dosage.

The side effects of neuroleptics have become so universal in their occurrence that there is a tendency to view them as part of the clinical condition itself. This misperception unnecessarily condemns patients to the agony of troublesome side effects and, in the case of tardive dyskinesia, perhaps an irreversible neurological disability.

Antidepressants and Lithium

Whereas, a few years ago, psychotherapy was the standard treatment for depression, large numbers of people now are managed with antidepressant medications.

Antidepressants generally fall into one of two chemical types: the tricyclics and the MAO-inhibitors. (Although some of the newer antidepressants are not strictly speaking tricyclics, they have similar effects and presumably have the same therapeutic mechanism of action.) The tricyclics (by far the most widely prescribed in this country) possess potent anticholinergic properties that, as previously mentioned, can precipitate symptoms of brain syndrome, especially in elderly persons. Both types of antidepressants can cause anxious agitation. In persons prone to cyclical mood swings, antidepressant medication may actually precipitate a full-blown, manic attack. Because many persons treated with these medications suffer from bipolar disorder, it is important to be aware of this reaction in order to intervene appropriately.

Lithium is a pharmacological mainstay in the management of bipolar disorder. This naturally occurring mineral has great efficacy in the treatment of acute manic attacks and is a preventive deterrent against future episodes. Unlike most other psychiatric medications, lithium requires close monitoring. As long as the blood level remains within a narrow therapeutic range, few troublesome effects are seen. When this range is exceeded, however, a host of disturbing and sometimes serious symptoms emerge.

Generally, the first manifestations of lithium toxicity are nausea, vomiting, or diarrhea. The person appears physically sick. Unfortunately, these early warning symptoms do not always develop. Instead, the clinician may confront an unexplained deterioration in the patient's ability to think clearly along with slurred speech and tremulousness. It is essential that the underlying culprit be recognized, because the margin of safety between therapeutic and toxic levels of lithium is relatively small.

An important drug interaction to remember concerning lithium is the toxicity-enhancing effect of certain diuretics used for treating hypertension. Lithium becomes toxic in the relative absence of sodium and potassium, minerals which often are depleted with the use of diuretics. For this reason, combined treatment (lithium and diuretic) requires close medical monitoring. Table 8.2 lists the most commonly prescribed antidepressants.

Minor Tranquilizers

The most widely prescribed medications in the United States are the benzodiazepine family of drugs used primarily to treat anxiety. Although relatively safe (especially when compared to the barbiturates) these drugs do have certain troublesome effects. Many benzodiazepines are long-acting. They (or their active metabolites) remain in the body for extended periods. Thus, if the same dose is taken day after day, a gradual accumulation results and the individual begins to feel drowsy, slowed down, depressed, and

TABLE 8.2 Antidepressants

Tricyclics		MAO-Inhibitors	
imipramine	(Tofranil®)	isocarboxazide	(Marplan®)
amitriptyline	(Elavil®)	phenelzine	(Nardil®)
doxepin	(Sinequan®)	tranylcypromine	(Parnate®)
desipramine	(Norpramin®)		

perhaps confused. These symptoms are intensified by alcohol. Rarely, individuals treated with the benzodiazepines will experience an opposite, "paradoxical" reaction, characterized by restlessness and agitation, or even rage.

Overall, the most serious problem associated with antianxiety agents is the addiction which develops with long and heavy usage. In these cases sudden stopping of the drug produces a dramatic withdrawal reaction with agitation, tremulousness and sometimes even psychosis. Given the increased use of high doses of alprazolam (Xanax®) in the treatment of panic attacks, it can be anticipated that benzodiazepine withdrawal will become an increasing problem. Table 8.3 contains a selective list of benzodiazepines.

Later in this chapter, we will consider in greater detail the clinical features of drug withdrawal.

GENERAL PRESCRIPTION MEDICATIONS

Antihypertensives and Cardiac Medications

High blood pressure medications have considerable potential for producing adverse mental effects. The chemical depletion or inactivation of the body's own catecholamines, while helping to lower blood pressure, may simultaneously cause depression. In fact, the first modern tranquilizer—rauwolfia—was accidentally discovered after it was recognized that persons treated for hypertension with this substance experienced a calming influence (an effect that with time, unfortunately, evolved into depression). Reserpine (a derivative of rauwolfia) is still used today in the treatment of hypertension.

Methyldopa (Aldomet®) is a popular antihypertensive which also causes depression, sometimes combined with symptoms of brain syndrome. The

TABLE 8.3 Benzodiazepines (Selected list)

diazepam	(Valium®)
chlordiazepoxide	(Librium®)
triazolam	(Halcione®)
alprazolam	(Xanax®)
oxazepam	(Serax®)
lorazepam	(Ativan®)

risk of this adverse reaction appears to be heightened when methyldopa is used in combination with haloperidol.

Diuretics have been used extensively to treat hypertension. As I mentioned, due to the tendency to deplete the body of potassium, prolonged use of diuretics can cause depression and fatigue. The same problem turns up in bulimics who, while using diuretics for a different reason, become depressed secondary to potassium loss.

Propranolol (Inderal®), and a host of other beta-adrenergic blocking drugs, has been around for some time. It also is used in the treatment of hypertension and angina pectoris as well as migraine. Depression is commonly a troublesome unintended consequence, as is sexual impotence in men. Less frequently, visual hallucinations, catatonia, and brain syndrome result.

Anti-inflammatory Drugs

Steroids have magical effects on certain diseases, especially those involving chronic inflammation—such as seen in rheumatoid arthritis and ulcerative colitis. Unfortunately, the powerful anti-inflammatory action of steroids causes severe physical and mental side effects when these medications are used extensively. Manic behavior—psychotic in intensity—can be induced by steroids, usually evolving out of the general euphoria experienced to some degree by most individuals placed on large doses.

In contrast, cases of profound depression with hallucinations have been described in association with Indocin® (indomethacin), a nonsteroidal, anti-inflammatory drug widely used in the treatment of rheumatoid arthritis. A non-steroidal, anti-inflammatory medication (ibuprofen) is now available without a prescription for treatment of pain or fever. Regular use may cause depression in susceptible individuals, particularly when taken in large doses.

When the Canadian Olympic track star, Ben Johnson, was stripped of his 100-meter gold medal at the Summer Olympics in Seoul, South Korea, a fact long known to athletes all over the world was flashed to the public:

Anabolic steroid use has become commonplace in the sports world, involving both professional and amateur athletes alike, particularly those engaged in power sports where brute strength is critical. (Although these drugs cannot be obtained legally without a prescription, they are readily available on a thriving black market.) "Stacking" is a common practice in which several steroids are used in sequence to achieve an optimal result; this practice also minimizes the chances that these drugs will be detected when drug testing is performed at competition time.

There is no doubt that anabolic steroids significantly increase muscle strength. The athletes who use them are usually quite knowledgeable about their strength-enhancing effects, but much less aware of the adverse consequences. Long-term use of anabolic steroids can damage the liver and heart. These drugs can also cause striking changes in mood and thought (Pope & Katz, 1987).

Two Harvard researchers interviewed 41 bodybuilders and football players who had used anabolic steroids. Thirteen of them reported manic-like symptoms, including hyperactivity, overinflated self-esteem, and grandiose and reckless behavior. One athlete bought a $17,000 sportscar. When he stopped taking the drug, he realized that he couldn't make the payments and was forced to sell the car. During a second manic episode, a year later, he impulsively purchased another expensive sportscar (*Discover,* 1988).

A second athlete became firmly convinced of his own invincibility while on anabolic steroids. To prove the point, he arranged for one of his friends to videotape him driving a car into a tree at 40 miles per hour!

In this same study, five athletes reported psychotic episodes. One had auditory hallucinations for five weeks; another developed paranoid delusions about his friends stealing from him. The psychotic symptoms disappeared when the steroids were stopped.

Serious depression has been reported by persons coming off of anabolic steroids. One 23-year-old body builder who had regularly taken four kinds of steroids told his doctor that he did not think he could stop because of the miserable depression and fatigue he experienced. Sure enough, one week off the steroids, the depression had become so great, he resumed taking them (*Los Angeles Times,* 1988).

Miscellaneous Medications

Stimulant medications are important in the management of asthma and other chronic respiratory diseases, such as bronchitis; and, despite their questionable effectiveness in achieving sustained weight loss, stimulants are prescribed as diet pills. These drugs can cause restlessness, irritability, insomnia and, with prolonged use, the insidious onset of paranoid psychosis.

Similar stimulant preparations are sold over-the-counter as "appetite suppressants." Their potential for adverse reactions is the same as for prescription diet pills. We will consider stimulants and their potential for inducing serious mental dysfunction at greater length in the section on street drugs.

Phenytoin (Dilantin®) is an effective anticonvulsant taken by many patients with seizure disorders. Its efficacy depends on the maintenance of an adequate blood level, which—if exceeded by only a small degree—leads to gross incoordination, mental dullness, and hallucinations. In addition, by interfering with the intestinal absorption of folic acid, phenytoin can cause brain syndrome along with diminished sensation and muscle strength.

The discovery of levodopa as a treatment for Parkinson's disease was a major breakthrough in what until that time had been a rather hopeless situation. A sizeable percentage of persons with this degenerative disease respond well to levodopa. Unfortunately, psychiatric side-effects are common. In a group of 88 patients with Parkinson's disease maintained on levodopa, roughly 50% experienced some form of psychiatric symptom during a year of treatment. Paranoid delusions, without confusion or disorientation, occurred in 9% of the patients. Roughly 3% developed symptoms of brain syndrome (Klawans, Moskovitz, Navsieda, & Weiner, 1979). Over time, levodopa treatment also leads to what is referred to as the "on–off" phenomenon in which the patient's parkinsonism periodically kicks back in momentarily with a marked slowing of movements. It is a frustrating aspect of levodopa treatment.

Cimetidine (Tagamet®) and ranitidine (Zantac®) are histamine (H_2 receptor) antagonists that drastically reduce gastric acidity. These drugs have revolutionized the medical treatment of gastrointestinal ulcer disease. This accounts for the meteoric rise in their usage worldwide. Particularly in older people, these anti-ulcer drugs cause depression, confusion, and visual hallucinations. There are also reports of impotence and loss of sexual interest thought to result from the blocking of androgenic hormones.

The clinician should also be alert to the adverse mental effects seen with two popular pain medications, propoxyphene (Darvon®) and pentazocine (Talwin®). Propoxyphene is widely prescribed for headache and minor pain. Chemically, it is related to the narcotic, methadone, and has proven capable of producing addiction and severe withdrawal reactions after prolonged use. Certain people react to even small doses with psychosis. Similarly, this reaction has been described in persons taking pentazocine.

Newer Drugs

The use of skin patches to deliver drugs *transdermally* has become common practice. For example, for the prevention of motion sickness, flat circular discs about the size of quarters are impregnated with scopolamine. This adhesive "patch" is placed behind a person's ear, where it provides sustained release of scopolamine targeted specifically at the vestibular apparatus. The theory is that this will cause fewer unwanted side effects. Unfortunately, this is not always true, particularly among the elderly.

> A 77-year-old woman, shortly after arriving for a vacation at a holiday resort, became confused and seemed to forget where she was. She was hospitalized, after which her symptoms rapidly cleared. No cause could be found.
> She was discharged and resumed her vacation. At the end of two weeks she returned home, where she immediately had a repeat episode of confusion and memory loss and, once again, was hospitalized. As on the first occasion, she quickly recovered. This time a more detailed history revealed that she had used a transdermal scopolamine patch to prevent car sickness on her way *to* and *from* the resort where she had vacationed. She was diagnosed as having suffered scopolamine delirium. (Rozzini, Inzoli, & Trabucchi, et al., 1988)

In this era of organ transplantation, cyclosporine—a drug which suppresses the immune system—has become life saving through its ability to prevent tissue rejection. In addition to its immunosuppressive action, in certain patients, it has caused complex visual hallucinations (Katirii, 1987).

Bromocriptine (Parlodel®) is an ergot derivative (as is LSD) with potent dopamine-like effects. It is used to prevent lactation in mothers who have just given birth; and, also, to restore normal menses in 89–90% of women with hyperprolactinemia. Its dopamine action is useful in the treatment of Parkinson's disease to ameliorate the marked swings ("on–off" phenome-

TABLE 8.4 Street Drugs (Selected list)

"Uppers"

"Speed" (methamphetamine)
"Bennies" (amphetamine)
"Coke" or "Crack" (cocaine)

Hallucinogens

LSD (lysergic acid diethylamide)
PCP (phencyclidine)
"Buttons" (psilocybin)

"Downers"

"Barbs" or "Reds" (barbiturates)
"Booze" (alcohol)
"Crank" (heroin)

non) that develop after extended treatment with levodopa. Bromocriptine can cause delusions, visual hallucinations, hypersexuality, and manic behavior.

Recombinant DNA technology holds the promise of creating a new generation of natural drugs. The interferons, for example, are a class of naturally occurring antiviral agents. These substances are now produced in large quantities and used in the treatment of AIDS and chronic viral hepatitis. In one study of patients treated with interferon for hepatitis, roughly one out of five developed psychological changes, including irritability, depression, extreme emotional lability, paranoia, and confusion (Renault, et al., 1987).

STREET DRUGS

The street scene is a constantly evolving drama. Today's favorite drugs give way to tomorrow's. Many street drugs are readily synthesized in backyard laboratories and thus become widely available. As there are no required quality controls in the illegal production of homemade psychoactive substances, the most recent batch may not be precisely the same as the one before it. What is in the "bag" may not even be the desired drug. There is also widespread adulteration of drugs after they are synthesized. The active drug is mixed with a lower-priced substance to maximize the overall profit margin. The effect on the unknowing user can be highly unpredictable.

Given these confounding aspects of the world of street drugs, the clinician is well advised to supplement patient histories with careful clinical observation because the patient may not know what he has taken or, if he does, may not be willing to divulge this information. The patient's behavior may be the clinician's best clue. Physical manifestations of street drugs often provide compelling evidence for a drug-induced mental problem: changes in pupil size, deviations in vital signs, slurred speech, or motor incoordination. Street drugs can be categorized roughly into three groups: stimulants ("uppers"), depressants ("downers"), and hallucinogens. See Table 8.4 for a selected list of specific substances.

"Uppers"

Uppers are best typified by the amphetamines and cocaine (crack). These drugs produce an energized euphoria with heightened activity, rapid speech, grandiosity, and sometimes belligerence. Because the stimulents trigger the sympathetic nervous system, the person's eyes are usually widely dilated and the pulse and blood pressure elevated. From a clinical perspective, an "upper trip" may appear like a manic episode, but the physiological changes are usually more prominent when the euphoria is drug-induced. If the drugs have been injected, track marks on the arms and legs help confirm the drug-related nature of the problem.

Chronic use of stimulants, particularly high doses, leads from increasing suspiciousness to paranoid psychosis, virtually indistinguishable from paranoid schizophrenia. This clinical presentation usually does not include the characteristic physiological changes, because these effects disappear as the body gradually adapts. The cognitive deficits of brain syndrome are *not* usually a part of amphetamine psychosis; in fact, an unusual degree of mental clarity may be preserved in this paranoid psychotic condition.

Due to the appetite-suppressing quality of stimulants, extended use may also lead to considerable weight loss so that the person's clothes no longer fit properly. The emergence of paranoid delusions in a person who has a history of trying to lose weight should always suggest the possibility of stimulant psychosis.

> After 2 months of unusual behavior, a 20-year-old woman was referred for psychiatric evaluation. She explained how she had felt increasingly "uptight." Upon initially meeting people, she strongly sensed she had met them previously. She related other strange events. She was certain that the students at her college were playing tricks on her—such as turning the clocks back. Her mother, she had come to believe, was planning to poison her.
>
> The woman explained these strange happenings as manifestations of a great struggle going on within herself involving the Holy Spirit, the Devil, and her own will. Each of these competing forces was expressed through a different language.
>
> During the interview, she appeared anxious. Although frankly delusional, she was fully oriented and coherent. She had no previous history of psychiatric problems and stated that she had been in excellent physical health. When questioned, she denied using street drugs, over-the-counter drugs, or prescribed medications. A diagnosis of acute paranoid schizophrenia was made and the woman was started on trifluoperazine® (Stelazine).
>
> Three weeks later, after her mental aberrations had subsided, she revealed to her therapist that she had been taking "diet pills" for three months.
>
> The revised diagnosis was "diet pill (stimulant) psychosis." (Hoffman, 1977)

All stimulants with extended use, can cause this type of paranoid psychosis.

One more thing about stimulants. There are cases that come to the clinician's attention after stimulant use has been discontinued, not as a typical withdrawal reaction (this does not occur with stimulants) but as severe depression. Unless the clinician is alert to the possibility of a *poststimulant depression,* he will become engaged in a fruitless search for nondrug-related, precipitating events.

Presently, cocaine (crack) is the stimulant of choice. Once considered a relatively safe recreational drug, it is now recognized as a dangerous and highly addictive substance. Due to its high cost, cocaine use was limited to the wealthier segments of the population until 1984 when a cheaper and more addicting version known as "crack," was introduced. Since then cocaine use has surged. The number of Americans who had tried cocaine increased from 5.4 million in 1974 to 25 million in 1985. Presently, it's estimated that more than 3 million Americans are addicted.

Cocaine use can cause medical problems ranging from the relatively mild discomforts of itching and coughing to life-threatening seizures, strokes, and cardiovascular collapse secondary to heart attack or arrhythmia.

It is not overstating the case to label cocaine *the great masquerader.* This popular stimulant produces a spectrum of psychological masquerades. The initial euphoria sometimes evolves into hyperexcitability and irritability, and can be mistaken for *manic behavior.* On other occasions the euphoria will take a different direction leading to severe anxiety, giving the clinical appearance of a *panic attack.* With prolonged use, the person may become increasingly suspicious until finally a *paranoid state* is reached, closely resembling schizophrenia.

Cocaine sometimes causes *brain syndrome,* usually of the rapid-onset variety, resulting in a clinical picture of delirium. *Hallucinosis* occurs. Serious *depression* may result when a user's supply is disrupted or an attempt is made to get off the drug.

Finally, due to cocaine craving, *sociopathy* and *criminal behavior* may become prominent as the person struggles to keep up with a habit that threatens to outstrip his or her financial resources.

After several days of hospitalization, a 27-year-old man, agitated and obsessed with his craving, left the hospital against his physician's advice.

He had been admitted for the psychiatric treatment of a paranoid psychosis. At the time of his admission, he appeared frail and underweight. He had had a string of serious cocaine binges, the maintenance of which consumed most of his time. His habit had left him penniless. In fact, he had financed his latest binge by selling his brother's car. His family considered this the last straw. They disowned him. When he left the hospital, he was on his own. (Manschreck, 1988)

Hallucinogens

A number of street drugs are capable of creating an array of perceptual distortions. Despite the name "hallucinogen," not all of these effects are actually hallucinations. Illusionary phenomena, for example, constitute a considerable part of the hallucinogenic experience. Hallucinations are only one of several kinds of perceptual distortions involving vision, taste, touch, smell, and self-awareness.

Synesthesias, in which one sensory form is perceived as another, are frequently experienced with hallucinogens. Music may sound like the taste of honey or the smell of lemon; or a strawberry may taste like the smell of vanilla or the sound of rain. Obviously such experiences when communicated to someone else (particularly a person who is not having the same experience and may not be aware that the person has taken a drug) can appear more psychotic than aesthetic.

A person under the influence of a hallucinogen is strongly influenced by factors other than the drug itself. The setting, the prevailing mood, and the nature of the relationship with other participants all contribute to the overall effect. Given the wrong mix, drug encounters can become extremely frightening and can quickly evolve into severe panic or paranoia. In other instances the individual may respond by becoming immobilized and mute, leading the unsuspecting clinician to a premature diagnosis of catatonic schizophrenia.

Many of the commonly used hallucinogens cause observable physiological changes, such as widely dilated pupils and elevations in pulse and blood pressure. This is not, however, a consistent finding.

Flashbacks plague a small percentage of persons who have taken hallucinogens; their specific cause is unknown. Days, weeks, sometimes even months or years after, a sudden fragmentary episode reminiscent of the actual drug experience erupts. Usually the flashback lasts no more than a few seconds and then disappears. The frequency of these attacks is quite variable, but usually with time they decrease and eventually disappear. Unaware of their origin, an individual may become quite troubled and begin to suspect he is losing his mind. The clinician, hearing a flashback described, may mistakenly suspect an impending functional psychosis.

Phencyclidine (PCP) is one of the most widely available hallucinogens, due mainly to the ease and cheapness with which it is made. The drug is both a potent analgesic and anesthetic agent that creates a kind of chemical sensory deprivation when taken in large doses. Bizarre, "spaced-out" behavior with a predilection for unprovoked violence characterizes PCP bad trips. There may be long periods of a blank, dazed expression and frozen posture. When the person does move, he is usually unsteady on his feet.

There is a tendency not to speak; and responses to any kind of stimulation are reduced. The symptoms of ROBS are often present, with dramatic swings in consciousness.

Unlike many other hallucinogens, PCP does not produce dilated pupils; there is, however, a characteristic up-and-down and side-to-side jerkiness of the eyes, known as nystagmus. Nystagmus is not specific to PCP intoxication. It is seen in other drug intoxications and in a variety of neurological conditions.

"Downers"

Alcohol is the prototype downer drug. Downers create a loosening of inhibitions and a sense of well-being. With large doses, the pleasant sensations give way to depression, decreased awareness, drowsiness, loss of consciousness, and sometimes coma and death. Numerous depressant substances are available. Considerable diversion into the black market occurs.

Downer abuse, typically, is denied. Recognition requires an index of suspicion and careful observation. The intoxicated person may be unsteady and have slurred speech. It is important to remember that downers are not used exclusively by the so-called drug culture. There is extensive use of these substances throughout the adult population.

Alcohol, the king of downers, is such a pervasive part of the social scene that often it is not even perceived as a drug. The fact is, it is the most extensively used drug in this country. The emotional and behavioral concomitants of chronic alcohol abuse—depression, anxiety, and suspiciousness—are frequently mistaken for psychological problems. Tell-tale signs, such as absenteeism, automobile accidents, and declining job or school performance are important indirect indicators of alcoholism. Family problems and other personal conflicts sometimes obscure the underlying problem. These should be seen as important, but secondary problems.

Persons suffering from alcoholism are not immune to other diseases; in fact, they experience a much higher incidence of serious organic conditions. These include subdural hematomas, hypoglycemia, liver disease, and several forms of cancer. Failure to suspect a serious medical problem masked by drunkenness is an all-too-common clinical mistake.

Alcohol potentiates most psychoactive drugs, including antidepressants, neuroleptics, minor tranquilizers, and particularly, other downers. In combination with these drugs, alcohol can cause an overdose condition, manifesting as confusion and drowsiness. In more tragic instances, such a combination becomes an unintentional cause of death.

DRUG WITHDRAWAL

Certain drugs create tolerance; that is, with extended use, increasing amounts are required to achieve the same effect. This is a defining characteristic of physically addicting substances. These drugs include barbiturates, analgesics, heroin, minor tranquilizers, and alcohol. The amount of time required to develop tolerance varies tremendously from one drug to another. Whereas with heroin or morphine tolerance ensues within days or weeks, alcohol tolerance occurs over a period of years. The end result, however, is the same.

The brain adapts to the effects of addicting drugs. Ironically, it is this adaptation that leaves the person susceptible to withdrawal reactions. When the drug is suddenly stopped after extended usage and the brain (in the case of downers) is no longer under this suppressing influence, "overshoot" occurs due to the increased neuronal activity that had arisen as an adaptation to the drug. In this sense drug withdrawal can be viewed as excessive neuronal activity giving rise to mental and physical aberrations.

Drug withdrawals have four characteristic facets, although in any given case, one or more may fail to appear.

Agitation

In the initial phase, the person is tremulous and anxious, easily startled by noises or unexpected events. He looks ill and is in obvious discomfort.

Physiological Changes

There is a rapid pulse rate, elevations in blood pressure and temperature, and excessive sweating. (Such changes may also indicate a supervening infectious disease such as pneumonia. Withdrawal alone, however, can produce them.)

Cognitive and Perceptual Disruption

Perceptual distortions, although typically appearing after the onset of agitation and physiological changes, may be the initial manifestation of withdrawal.

Rapid-onset brain syndrome is common and can be accompanied by

paranoid delusions. Cognitive distortions typically begin with mispercep-
tions of things in the immediate environment (illusions) and then progress
to hallucinations. Hallucinated voices are often insulting and accusatory.
Visual hallucinations are commonplace. The perennial objects of alcohol
jokes—pink elephants and little green men—are *in fact* encountered by
persons in the throes of delirium tremens. The more severe the withdrawal
reaction, the more frightening the hallucinations. Snakes and spiders may
be seen crawling on the walls, the ceiling, or on the floor. Even more frightening, the individual may sense he is infested by bugs which no one else
can see.

With respect to cognitive disruption and psychosis, heroin withdrawal is a
notable exception. These symptoms are seldom seen. Physical flu-like
symptoms, characteristically, are much more prominent.

Seizures

Seizures occur in a relatively small percentage of appropriately treated
cases of drug withdrawals; but in untreated cases—particularly those involving downers—this complication is more frequent and can be life-threatening.

> A disheveled man in his fifties was found lying in an alleyway, grasping at
> his chest and complaining of pain. An ambulance was called, and the man
> was taken to the emergency room of a county hospital. He was found to have
> suffered a severe heart attack.
>
> Over the next two days, the patient's chest pain subsided. He was coopera-
> tive, fully oriented, and able to carry on a conversation. He denied any pre-
> vious history of serious illness, trauma, or alcohol consumption; but because
> he had smelled of alcohol on admission, his story was considered suspect.
>
> By the end of the second day, the patient had become agitated and was
> verbally abusive with hospital staff, quite different from his previous friendly
> and cooperative demeanor. That evening he was found standing in his bed,
> undaunted by the leads from the heart monitor and the I.V. going into his
> arm. He was sweating profusely and shouting out commands as though he
> were the captain of a ship and the immediate hospital surroundings an
> ocean-going vessel. Staff and other patients were addressed as ship person-
> nel. The man's eyes shifted about as though he were responding to visual
> hallucinations. He carried on conversations with imaginary persons, using
> graphic expletives and dramatic gestures. His pulse rate, blood pressure, and
> temperature were all elevated.
>
> For his own safety, the man was subdued and restrained in bed. Over the
> next 24 hours, despite aggressive treatment for delirium tremens, his condi-

tion failed to improve. His situation then became complicated by the onset of pneumonia. He quickly deteriorated, expiring on the fifth hospital day.

It was assumed that the man had been an alcoholic who had suffered a severe heart attack. When due to his hospitalization, he had suddenly stopped drinking, he had experienced a delirium tremens which, in combination with pneumonia, led to his death. (Taylor, 1980)

The clinical presentations of drug withdrawal are variable. The typical situation, much like the preceding case, involves a person brought in for treatment or confinement in jail because of severe inebriation. After the symptoms of intoxication subside, over the next 12 to 36 hours, the stage is set for withdrawal.

Clinicians sometimes dismiss the possibility of drug withdrawal if all the characteristic symptoms are not present or if it is clear that the person has not completely stopped using drugs or alcohol. This is a mistake. Drug withdrawal can manifest as a single symptom such as hallucination, and can develop after only a *reduction* in the amount of drug consumed. *Abstinence is not a necessary requirement for drug withdrawal.*

The severity of withdrawal reactions depends on the particular substance and the amount and duration of use. It is a widely held misconception that withdrawal from opiate drugs (such as heroin) is the most serious form of drug withdrawal. Not so. The death rate from cold turkey heroin withdrawals is extremely low; in contrast, withdrawal from barbiturates carries a significant mortality rate, even higher than that seen in alcoholic delirium tremens. Because the barbiturate addict frequently does not fit the stereotypical image of the "drugger," this potentially lethal condition is easily overlooked.

Finally, the clinician should be aware of what can be a particularly baffling form of drug withdrawal. Usually, the case involves a person who has ingested pills as a suicide attempt or is acutely intoxicated. The person is admitted to a treatment facility, "drunk." Unknown to the clinician, there has been an extensive history of substance abuse, frequently including mixed use of benzodiazepines, pain medications, and alcohol. As the immediate effects of the overdose wear off, the clinical condition begins to shift radically. Because the patient no longer has access to his or her supply of drugs, withdrawal symptoms begin to displace the initial clinical picture of intoxication. This shifting clinical presentation can leave the unsuspecting clinician quite bewildered.

Drug use is pervasive; it is epidemic. The clinician is well advised to maintain a high index of suspicion for drug-induced mental disorders.

REFERENCES

Ban, T. (1976). Drug interactions with psychoactive drugs. *Diseases of the Nervous System, 36,* 164–166.

Discover. (1988, September 8) Muscling in on Madness. p. 8.

Gelenberg, A., & Mandel, M. (1977). Catatonic reactions to high-potency neuroleptic drugs. *Archives of General Psychiatry, 34,* 947–950.

Granacher, R., & Baldessarini, R. (1975). Physostigmine. *Archives of General Psychiatry, 32,* 375–380.

Hall, R., Popkin, M., Stickney, S., & Gardner, D. (1978). Covert outpatient drug abuse: incidence and therapist recognition. *Journal of Nervous and Mental Disease, 1661,* 343–348.

Hoffman, B. (1977). Diet pill psychosis (letter). *Canadian Medical Journal, 116,* 351–355.

Juergens, S., & Morse, R. (1988). Alprazolam dependence in seven patients. *American Journal of Psychiatry, 145,* 625–627.

Katirii, M. (1987). Visual hallucinations and cyclosporine. *Transplantation, 43,* 768–769.

Klawans, H., Moskovitz, C., Navsieda, P., & Weiner, W. (1979). Levodopa-induced dopaminergic hypersensitivity in the pathogenesis of psychiatric and neurological disorders. *International Journal of Neurology, 13,* 225–236.

Los Angeles Times. (1988, September 5). Steroid Addiction Reported. Part II, p. 3.

Manschreck, T. (1988, August). Cocaine abuse, medical and psychopathologic effects. *Drug Therapy,* p. 26.

Meyers, B. (1988). Psychological misinterpretations in the diagnosis of acute dystonia. *Psychosomatics, 29,* 224–226.

Pope, H., & Katz, D. (1987). Bodybuilder's psychosis. *Lancet i,* 863.

Renault, P., Hoofnagle, J., Park, Y., Mullen, K., Peters, M., Jones, B., Rustgi, V., & Jones, A. (1987). Psychiatric complications of long-term interferon alpha therapy. *Archives of Internal Medicine, 147,* 1577–1580.

Rozzini, R., Inzoli, M., Trabucchi, M., et al. (1988). Delirium from transdermal scopolamine in an elderly woman. *Journal of the American Medical Association, 260,* 478.

Shader, R., & Greenblatt, D. (1971). Uses and toxicity of belladonna alkaloids in synthetic anticholinergics. *Seminars in Psychiatry, 3,* 449–476.

Siris, S. (1985). Three cases of akasthisia and "acting out". *Journal of Clinical Psychiatry, 46,* 395–397.

Taylor, R. (1980). Extracted from private clinical files.

Taylor, R., Maurer, J., & Tinklinberg, J. (1970). Management of "bad trips" in an evolving drug scene. *JAMA, 213,* 422–425.

Chapter 9

Somatization:
The Other Side of Things

Judge not according to appearance.   —St. John

Up to this point we have considered ways in which organic disorders masquerade as psychological problems. In this chapter we take up the reverse side of the coin: the translation of psychological conflicts into physical or somatic symptoms in the absence of underlying organic disease. This is called *somatization.* These conditions are listed in DSM-III-R as "Somatoform Disorders" (American Psychiatric Association, 1987).

You might be asking yourself how a consideration of somatization fits into the theme of this book. Because somatization presents clinically as "physical" symptoms, there would seem to be little risk of psychological masquerade. The problem is that, terms such as "psychosomatic" and "hysterical" are often applied too loosely. Anyone who complains of vague somatic symptoms in this age of pop psychology runs the risk of being labeled "psychosomatic."

This chapter reviews the usual patterns of somatization so that *atypical findings* will stand out. Confronted with "psychosomatic" cases, the clinician should confirm that appropriate medical evaluation has failed to find an organic cause and that there is a clinical history consistent with the somatization hypothesis. Clinicians should not fall into the trap of automatically construing vague physical symptoms as somatic expressions of psychological problems. You will recall in a study referred to earlier, of 85 persons initially diagnosed as suffering from hysteria, over one-third, in fact, turned out to have organic disease. It is a sobering reminder that somatization is not always what it seems to be. As we review the usual patterns of somatization, the essential findings will be described. When these are absent, the diagnosis of somatization must be considered highly tentative. It is much more important for a nonmedical psychotherapist to conclude confidently that "this is probably *not* a case of somatization" than to speculate that "this is a case of somatization." The latter should be left to those responsible for medical evaluation.

SIMPLE SOMATIZATION

From time to time most of us experience somatic symptoms without any demonstrable organic basis. Studies have shown that as many as 60–80% of healthy individuals during any given week report somatic complaints (Kellner, 1987). The various demands of day-to-day living have a way (not clearly understood) of becoming translated into somatic language. Perhaps it's merely a matter of being more aware of minor aches and pains that otherwise might be ignored; or, maybe it's that persons under stress react with greater muscle tension, resulting in vague somatic soreness or discomfort. Whatever the reason, many people who seek medical help suffer from somatization whose etiology is psychosocial.

Although somatic symptoms are characteristic of many organic diseases, when they are vague and ill-defined, often, they are expressions of *simple somatization*. The basic guideline for evaluating somatic complaints is this: Well-defined somatic symptoms of increasing severity and extended duration (more than a few days) always should be medically evaluated; and, the same is true of vague somatic symptoms if they fail to conform to the patterns that we will review in this chapter.

There are four essential characteristics of simple somatization. First, there should be no obvious organic basis (or strong suggestion of it) as would be the case in persons with a history of medical disease that can produce the current symptoms.

Second, the somatic complaints should occur in the contexts of a stressful life situation: perhaps a problem at work, marital difficulty, a personal loss, or a major life transition. Often when the stress is identified and openly discussed, simple somatization quickly resolves.

Temporariness is the third essential characteristic. The long-standing doctor joke—"Take two aspirin and call me in the morning"—plays on an important principle that physicians and other healers have taken advantage of for centuries: the body, given time, tends to heal itself psychologically as well as physically. This is certainly the case with simple somatization. Even if a stressful situation persists, the person gradually adapts and the severity of the somatic complaints diminishes. Typically, the clinical picture of simple somatization is not one of persistence or increasing severity; this is much more characteristic of organic disease.

Finally, somatization complaints are usually vague in nature. Even if encouraged to be more specific, the patient likely will have difficulty doing so. When a person describes a somatic symptom in specific detail, simple somatization is not the most likely explanation.

For the clinician considering somatic symptoms, the rule is this: *If somatic symptoms occur without identifiable stress, if they persist or intensify, or if they are specifically described, seriously consider organic disease.* (Also if the person has a history of organic disease with similar symptoms, a recurrence must be ruled out.)

One word of warning: what appears at first to be a vague complaint, with slight elaboration by the clinician often proves to be a specific physical symptom. Take fatigue. This common complain may serve as a projective test for clinicians, plunging them into premature conclusions: "Fatigued? Yes, well how long have you been depressed?"

Fatigue does not necessarily imply depression and certainly should not be equated with it. When a patient complains of fatigue, the clinician should encourage the person to explain.

CLINICIAN: "What do you mean when you say you feel fatigued?"
PATIENT: "Well, I don't have any energy."
CLINICIAN: "What makes you say you don't have any energy?"
PATIENT: "At any job, I can't carry the heavy containers . . . mainly seems to be my left arm. Guess I'm just getting old."

In the course of this short hypothetical exchange, the initial, vague-sounding complaint of "feeling fatigued" has been circumscribed as weakness in the left arm, a very specific physical symptom and probably not an expression of simple somatization.

Consider a second symptom.

PATIENT: "I'm not my old self; I'm just not well."
CLINICIAN: "Not well?"
PATIENT: "Yeah, I hardly even get out of the house."
CLINICIAN: "Why not?"
PATIENT: "I can't walk more than a few steps without getting out of breath. Can't even make it up the stairs at home without being winded."

What is initially described as "I'm just not my old self; I'm just not well," with brief clarification, translates into: "I get completely out of breath." Breathlessness is a physical symptom commonly seen in various heart and lung conditions. It deserves a complete medical evaluation.

Organic diseases causing persons to feel apathetic, fatigued, breathless, or weak can easily be misinterpreted as psychosomatic conditions. Anemia is a good example. This is a common medical problem, especially among women. The most frequent cause is iron deficiency, which often develops after the cumulative loss of iron from heavy menstrual periods. Other conditions, such as ulcers, hemorrhoids, and certain internal cancers, also produce chronic blood loss and anemia. Regardless of the precise etiology, anemia can lead to certain core symptoms: pallor, fatigue, lassitude, and breathlessness on mild exertion. Diagnostic mistakes arise when the fatigue, lassitude, and reduced activity are construed prematurely as instances of "depression with somatic overlay." Vague somatic symptoms should always be pursued with clarifying questions.

Hyperparathyroidism, although not nearly as common as anemia, can also masquerade as somatization. The parathyroid glands (small, pea-shaped nodules located in the neck adjacent to the thyroid gland) play a central role in the body's regulation of calcium. In hyperparathyroidism, an excessive amount of parathyroid hormone is released, causing high concentrations of calcium in the blood and urine. The calcium precipitates in the kidneys, causing stones that produce shifting abdominal and back pain as they pass from the body. In addition, complaints of generalized aches and pains arise as calcium is rapidly mobilized from the bones. Approximately 25% of patients with hyperparathyroidism develop peptic ulcer, providing yet another kind of somatic complaint. When such complaints are combined with muscle weakness, lethargy, and depression, a "psychosomatic" diagnosis may become irresistible.

> Apathetic, depressed and losing her strength, a 68-year-old widow explained her deteriorating condition as the product of loneliness. For four years she had also suffered from intermittent, upper-abdominal discomfort.
>
> After being evaluated by her internist, the woman was seen by a consulting psychiatrist who diagnosed her as moderately depressed. During the course of a medical evaluation, however, a duodenal ulcer was discovered during a radiographic study of her gastrointestinal tract.
>
> Further investigation showed an elevated serum calcium level (12mg/100ml), leading to a diagnosis of hyperparathyroidism. At surgery a parathyroid adenoma (a benign tumor) was removed. The woman recovered without complication and experienced prompt healing of her ulcer. Her symptoms of lethargy, weakness, and depression resolved without additional therapy. (Martin, 1979)

Here we have illustrated the importance of distinguishing muscle weakness form complaints of lethargy, apathy, or fatigue. Until proven otherwise, muscle weakness should be considered a neurological problem. There is a tendency on the part of therapists to view somatic complaints as peripheral concerns. It's an unsound practice. Somatic symptoms are often telltale clues to masquerading organic problems. If ignored, the underlying causative condition may be overlooked. The syndrome of hyperventilation serves as a good example, illustrating the pitfalls of ignoring somatic symptoms.

Hyperventilation syndrome is an episodic organic condition, typically evolving out of a state of psychological anxiety. As the anxiety builds, the person starts to overbreathe; the breathing becomes deeper and more rapid. Symptoms result from the blowing off of excessive carbon dioxide, disrupting the essential balance between oxygen and carbon dioxide. This causes an alkaline shift in the blood pH level. Among other changes, this pH shift produces a sense of apprehension, setting into motion a vicious cycle leading to more anxiety. Various somatic complaints emerge. Lightheadedness and numbness around the mouth and in the fingers and toes are common, as are breathlessness, chest pain, and headache. Rarely, in severe cases, the person may develop muscle spasms that twist the wrists and ankles. Hallucinations sometimes occur.

When the entire spectrum of symptoms is present, the organic nature of hyperventilation is usually obvious. In more typical cases, however, the clinician encounters an extremely anxious person who may relate a plausible reason for being upset. The somatic symptoms may be understated by the patient, or if commented on, neglected by the interviewer. A point to remember is that once a person has overbreathed to the extent of causing symptoms, continuous rapid breathing is no longer required to sustain the chemical imbalance. A few deep, sighing breaths periodically will do the trick.

> Accompanied by her boyfriend, a 22-year-old woman sought medical care at a local hospital emergency room for what she thought was a heart attack.
> Frightened and anxious, she complained of shortness of breath and chest pain. She also described a tingling sensation around her mouth as well as lightheadedness. Her symptoms had developed soon after she had discovered that her boyfriend had been with another woman. (Dubousky & Weissberg, 1978)

If a person is hyperventilating, a reduction in the rate and depth of breathing will quickly ameliorate the symptoms. The patient should be encouraged to relax and breathe more slowly. Sometimes the person will be too anxious to follow this direction. If so, he or she can be instructed to breathe into and out of a brown paper bag for a few minutes. This time-honored technique ensures the rebreathing of carbon dioxide. The result: a dramatic disappearance of symptoms.

The hyperventilation syndrome should be suspected in all cases of acute anxiety, particularly when associated with its characteristic complaints. But this clinical picture can also result from specific diseases. In one study of 30 patients with hyperventilation, seven were found to have complicating organic disorders (Pincus & Tucker, 1974). Although it is possible that in certain of these cases the symptoms arose out of anxiety concerning the physical disease, in most instances the disease itself caused the problem. This possibility should be considered if symptoms of hyperventilation do not come under control easily or if they tend to recur after only brief periods of relief.

Hyperventilation sometimes occurs in conjunction with *panic disorder*, a variant of generalized anxiety. Panic disorder is seen most commonly in individuals who are genetically susceptible, as evidenced by increased concordance in identical twins and considerably greater risk for anxiety disorder among relatives.

As for the attacks themselves, they usually first appear in young adulthood. Characteristically, the person abruptly feels anxious for no apparent reason. Somatic symptoms are usually prominent, including several of the following: breathlessness, palpitations, headache, sweating, smothering sensation, faintness, light-headedness, chest pain, tremulousness, and numbness and tingling (particularly around the mouth, fingers, and toes). Many patients sense that they are having a heart attack. It is not unusual for panic attack victims to show up in emergency rooms or urgent care centers; and, eventually, some are subjected to invasive cardiac testing. One study of 33 cardiac catheterization patients who turned out to have normal coronary arteries found that one-third fit the criteria for panic disorder (Mukerjiv & Alpert, 1987).

Subjectively, panic attack patients are extremely frightened and often feel that they may die. Some become negatively conditioned to the places where the attacks take place. As a result, afterward, they avoid returning to the site. Gradually, as these phobias build up, their lives become progressively restricted, until in some cases, the person becomes housebound (agoraphobic).

Of theoretical interest, after intravenous infusion of sodium lactate solution, 50% of panic disorder patients experience an attack as compared to 9% of persons who have no history of anxiety or panic disorder (Cowley & Roy-Byrne, 1987). The etiological significance of this response is not clear, but this biological marker along with the evidence for genetic loading strongly suggests a biological basis for panic disorder. Additionally, 80% of patients respond favorably to antidepressant medication. Within four weeks of continuous treatment, roughly half of patients are symptom-free (Klerman, 1988).

Panic attacks, however, are not always the product of panic disorder. They can be mimicked by other medical conditions. The most likely candidates are hyperthyroidism, cardiac arrhythmias, complex partial seizures, hypoglycemia, and stimulant drug use (including caffeine). This point is well illustrated in the following case.

One week after she and her husband had resigned as motel managers, a 55-year-old woman experienced severe anxiety. Along with her anxiousness, she had difficulty breathing, tightness in her throat, and a feeling of impending doom. She said that she was acutely aware of her heart beating and felt things becoming unreal. The first episode was followed by a steady stream of similar occurrences.

Her husband said that during these episodes she was difficult to understand (on occasion she had bitten her tongue) and seemed unaware of what was going on around her. Sometimes she became agitated and fell to the ground. The attacks lasted anywhere from a few minutes to an hour.

Finally, the woman sought help at an outpatient psychiatric clinic. She related how four times over the past three months she had been taken by paramedic ambulance to emergency rooms. Each time, her evaluation turned up nothing more than mild hypertension.

A Doppler flow study of her carotid arteries was normal. She had experienced a significant weight loss: 60 pounds during a three-month period (from 280 to 220 pounds). She had no history of psychiatric illness. On examination, the patient appeared anxious but was fully alert and coherent. She reported difficulty concentrating and suffered from moderate depression, including crying spells and feelings of low self-worth. She also had become afraid to leave her house, demanding that her husband stay with her at all times.

The patient was given a diagnosis of "agoraphobia with panic attacks and concurrent depression." She was treated with imipramine 50 mg, increasing to 150 mg over a two-week period, and diazepam 5 mg four times a day. Within a short time, her anxiety disappeared. For three weeks the woman had no further attacks.

Her physician then received a telephone call from her husband telling him that she had developed right-sided weakness. Later, in the emergency room, this weakness was interpreted as a hysterical reaction; but when it progressed in severity, she was admitted to a psychiatric unit. There she was examined by two residents in neurology. They too thought that her anxiety and weakness were psychological!

For legal reasons, she was given an EEG and CT scan which revealed a left-sided, fronto-parietal mass (glioblastoma multiforme). Following surgical removal, her panic attacks disappeared. (Dietch, 1984)

In retrospect, it was thought that this woman's "panic attacks" were most likely complex partial seizures related to rapid tumor growth. The major clinical tipoffs were: speech disturbance, biting of her tongue, falling to the ground and loss of awareness during these episodes. Also, at age 55, she was considerably older than patients having their first panic attack.

TABLE 9.1 **Essential Characteristics of Simple Somatization**

Has no obvious organic basis
Occurs in association with increased life stress
Fails to persist beyond the stress period
Manifests as nonspecific, vague complaints

While in many cases, panic disorder is overlooked and persons suffering from it are unnecessarily subjected to invasive diagnostic procedures, it is important to keep in mind that as this diagnosis becomes more "popular," there is the danger of applying it prematurely. (This woman was examined by eight physicians before the correct diagnosis was made.)

Although somatic expressions of psychosocial stress are common, the clinician should guard against interpreting all cases of vague somatic complaints as simple somatization, particularly in the absence of the essential characteristics listed in Table 9.1.

BRIQUET'S SYNDROME (HYSTERIA OR SOMATIZATION DISORDER)

Due to the vagueness of the term, "hysteria," its usefulness has been questionable. For this reason, a replacement—"Briquet's syndrome," after the French physician who described a striking form of somatization in 1859—has been suggested (Woodruff, Goodwin & Guse, 1974). This syndrome typically begins during the teen years with the emergence of multiple physical complaints that have no organic basis; nevertheless, various diagnoses, hospitalizations, and treatments (including surgery) accumulate, along with an ever-growing list of discarded physicians. The person with Briquet's syndrome becomes compulsively preoccupied with ill health; complaining about physical symptoms becomes a way of life.

Exaggerating and overdramatizing symptoms is an essential aspect of Briquet's syndrome, as is a history of significant interpersonal conflict, particularly of a sexual nature. One researcher has even suggested that this diagnosis is highly questionable when a satisfactory sexual life is reported by the individual.

The clinician should not equate multiple somatic symptoms with Briquet's syndrome. It is the total absorption by the person—continuing over years—in their physical symptoms and the professionals from whom they seek help. People with this severe form of somatization invariably have thick medical charts and therapy records.

For several years, an unemployed 31-year-old divorced man had complained of multiple psychiatric and somatic symptoms. During a divorce, he had become depressed and had (on several occasions) disappeared for extended periods. Each time, upon his return, his memory for what had transpired was clouded.

The man had been admitted to a psychiatric hospital nine times. Each time his inpatient treatment was disrupted by numerous diagnostic procedures to investigate his multiple somatic complaints. No organic basis had ever been found.

There was an extensive medical history dating back to the age of 12, when he had been hospitalized for abdominal pain, initially thought to be appendicitis. On further evaluation, he was discharged without treatment. Five years later he was hospitalized again, this time for long-lasting headaches. No organic basis could be determined. At age 30 a recurrent bout of abdominal pain led to another round of exhaustive but unproductive medical workups.

More recently, he was operated on for gallstones, but at the time of surgery, the gallbladder was found to be normal. Over the years, this man had been extensively evaluated for endocrine, cardiac, and respiratory problems and a variety of gastrointestinal complaints. No organic pathology was found. (On one occasion, however, at age 24, this man did have severe pain from renal stones.)

Upon being interviewed, he alleged the current existence of more than 30 different physical symptoms, many of which were described in exaggerated terms. For example, when asked if he had experienced fatigue, he responded: "Yes. Sometimes I have more energy than Carter has pills, but sometimes I don't have enough energy to pick up a pin."

He related a past history of considerable uncomfortableness and embarrassment about sex. After being exclusively homosexual between the ages of 16 and 21, he acceded to pressure from his mother and started seeing women. Soon thereafter he married. The relationship was marked by marital discord. He found himself indifferent to sex and impotent much of the time.

Mentally, he was oriented without delusions or hallucinations. He was described as "flamboyant," "enthusiastic," and "friendly." At times he was overly emotional, easily moved to tears or laughter without provocation. Surprisingly, he expressed a belief that most of his problems—mental and physical—had psychological causes. (Kaminsky & Slavney, 1976)

Although this case history of Briquet's syndrome contains the essential features—early onset, extensive number of somatic complaints, numerous normal medical evaluations, dramatic presentations, and a history of chronic sexual dissatisfaction—it also includes certain notable aberrations. First, the patient is a man. By far, most cases of Briquet's syndrome occur in women; obviously, there are exceptions. Second, this patient seemed to have an awareness of the psychological nature of his problem. Perhaps more extensive interviewing would have shown this to be deceptive, but to the degree that it was present, it is an unexpected finding. Much more characteristic would have been total unwillingness to entertain the possibility of a psychological explanation.

One other aspect of this case is worth emphasizing: the occurrence, in conjunction with Briquet's syndrome, of renal stones, a bona fide organic disease. *People who somatize sometimes become physically ill.* A point to keep in mind.

Certain diseases, by attacking multiple organ systems, precipitate multiple complaints and can be confused with Briquet's syndrome. Take the following case:

> Shortly after the aircraft manufacturing firm for which he worked began to lay off employees, a 32-year-old aeronautical engineer, father of three, reluctantly consulted his family physician, complaining of transient episodes of double vision, dizziness, leg weakness, and "tingling" sensations in his legs over a three-month period.
>
> During this same time the man had been involved in two minor automobile accidents while driving alone in his car. On both occasions he had sustained minor lacerations.
>
> As for his personal life, his marriage of 11 years was described as good. Other than infrequent arguments with his wife about money, they seemed to get along well.
>
> The patient had been in excellent health. He denied ever having fainting spells, convulsions, paralysis, or problems with speech. Two years prior, his father (with whom he had been quite close) had died from a stroke.
>
> The man was intelligent. His memory was excellent. Early in the interview he expressed the idea that his symptoms might be caused by stress over the threat of losing his job. His physical examination, including a careful neurological assessment, revealed no abnormal findings. (Fuller, 1976)

If the facts of this case are carefully considered, Briquet's syndrome is a highly unlikely possibility.

In his early thirties, this patient had no previous history of somatization. Furthermore, rather than rushing to the doctor with a dramatic elaboration of symptoms, he had delayed for three months and even then had sought out his family physician reluctantly. His 11-year marriage suggested a degree of interpersonal stability, and his willingness to consider the possibility of a psychological explanation suggested considerable psychological awareness. Based on these findings, a psychiatric consultant who had been asked to evaluate the case concluded that there was strong evidence *against* this being hypochondriasis or a hysterical conversion reaction. The patient was discharged without a definitive diagnosis. A few months later, he developed full-blown neurological symptoms including partial paralysis and sensory loss. He was diagnosed as having multiple sclerosis.

Multiple sclerosis (MS) is a degenerative neurological disease of undetermined etiology. It causes patchy destruction of the nerve coverings, thereby producing a kind of short circuiting throughout the nervous system. The symptoms are diverse: they may include sensory changes, visual disturbances, selective weakness, difficulty speaking, and increased emotionality. Symptoms abruptly arise and then diminish or disappear after a short while, only to recur again months or even years later. Initially, temporary deficits in vision and other sensory modalities may be the only symptoms; with time, however, additional neurological deficits develop and gradually become more severe. To date, no curative treatment has been discovered.

Given its diverse and shifting symptomatology, multiple sclerosis is easily mistaken for somatization.

A group of diseases collectively known as "autoimmune diseases" attack different parts of the body, creating a mystifying array of symptoms. Autoimmune diseases are thought to result from a "memory lapse" in the body's own immune system. Early in embryonic development, the immune system memorizes the difference between the body's own cells and foreign invaders such as bacteria and viruses. The ability to make this distinction allows the immune system to selectively seek out and destroy agents of disease, without doing damage to the body itself.

For reasons not fully understood, in autoimmune diseases the immune system's ability to distinguish between "self" and "not self" fails. This essential surveillance system becomes confused and attacks the person's own body as though it were a foreign invader. The result: A spectrum of degenerative diseases whose symptoms differ according to which of the body's organ systems are most assaulted. Either as a result of direct damage to the brain itself or as a manifestation of support system failure, mental symptoms are common in autoimmune diseases.

In a study of patients with an autoimmune disease—systemic lupus erythematosus (SLE)—medical researchers found that roughly one-fifth had psychiatric symptoms at some time during the course of the disease. A variety of intermittent somatic symptoms easily mistaken for somatization occurred. Joint pains (arthralgias) were found in 92% of cases; pleuritic pain in 54%, and fatigue and breathlessness in 32% (Feinglass, Arnett, Porsch, Zizic, & Steverns, 1976).

Cancer of the pancreas, often initially causes vague abdominal discomfort that may defy diagnosis. Even more confusing, this cancer is frequently associated with depression. Research psychiatrists found that one-third of patients (9 of 28) with pancreatic cancer met the diagnostic criteria for major depression. In comparison, no cases of depression were found in nine patients with stomach cancer (Joffe, Rubinow, Denicoff, Maher, & Sindelar, 1986). Although the exact mechanism is unknown, cancer of the pancreas has a special proclivity for causing depression; consequently, it is frequently (particularly early in the course of the disease) misinterpreted as a psychiatric condition. These patients often report an uncanny foreboding; a personal sense of impending doom. This emotional response can easily be dismissed as hysterical, and as the disease progresses other symptoms such as nausea, back pain, and weight loss may be ignored, overshadowed by the clinical picture of depression.

A 59-year-old woman with no previous history of mental illness developed insomnia, nervousness, and depression. She also complained of weakness, vague abdominal symptoms, and a striking loss of appetite, resulting in a 10-pound weight loss over four months.

Finally, she was admitted to a hospital for a medical workup. She gave a history of crying spells and depression. At one point she informed her doctor that she thought something terrible was about to happen to her.

A complete physical examination, including gastrointestinal studies, failed to reveal any organic disease. She was discharged with a diagnosis of neurasthenia and anxiety neurosis.

Two months later, after continued weight loss and abdominal pain, the woman was reexamined. A hard mass was detected in the upper left side of her abdomen. At surgery, carcinoma of the body of the pancreas was found; but, due to its advanced stage of growth, it was inoperable. The patient died at home a few weeks later. (Yaskin, 1931)

Abdominal discomfort, depression, and weight loss in a middle-aged or older person should make the clinician suspicious of pancreatic cancer. Whereas Briquet's syndrome seldom appears after the age of 30, cancer of the pancreas is rare before age 45. In the absence of the essential characteristics summarized in Table 9.2, the clinician should resist labeling symptoms as hysterical or Briquet's syndrome.

Although somewhat controversial, two other conditions should be considered when vague somatic complaints are found in conjunction with fatigue and depression. The first is fibromyalgia (fibrositis). Many rheumatologists say this is the most common condition they see in their practices. The patients complain of early morning stiffness, fatigue or exhaustion, and sleepiness (regardless of how many hours they sleep at night). At least 25% report depression and a sense of total exhaustion. When examined by a physician, they usually have points of tenderness, particularly over various bony prominences (Kirmayer, Robbins, & Kapusta, 1988).

The second condition is chronic mononucleosis (Epstein-Barr disease). A percentage of persons who develop infectious mononucleosis (caused by the Epstein-Barr herpes virus), afterward suffer recurrent bouts of fatigue, vague somatic complaints, depression, low-grade fever, and environmental

---

TABLE 9.2 Essential Characteristics of Briquet's Syndrome

Has no obvious organic basis

Presents as extensive number of somatic complaints (minimum 13)

Dates back to teens or early twenties

Includes extensive dramatic elaboration of symptoms

Has history of chaotic interpersonal relationships, particularly with respect to sexuality

---

allergies. These patients have elavated antibody titers to the Epstein-Barr virus. On the other hand, many individuals with similar antibody levels fail to report symptoms (Hellinger et al., 1988).

Both fibromyalgia and chronic mononucleosis are much more common among women than men. Although there are reports of favorable responses to low-dose antidepressant medication, much remains to be understood about these two conditions and their treatments.

CONVERSION DISORDER

Conversion disorder—also called hysterical conversion neurosis—refers to the sudden, dramatic appearance of a "neurological problem" that when fully evaluated is found to have no organic basis. Since the time of Freud, the most widely accepted explanation posits that this condition represents repressed psychological conflict translated into somatic language. The idea is that the conflict is more acceptable to the person expressed somatically than psychologically.

Unlike Briquet's syndrome, conversion disorder usually produces a single, prominent symptom (or symptom complex) rather than multiple diverse complaints and has an abrupt, explosive onset. Conversion disorder, however, can be superimposed on Briquet's syndrome; and like Briquet's syndrome, it is much more common in women. As shown in Table 9.3 conversion disorder can be divided into three clinical types.

In *loss of function* conversion, the deficit involves loss of movement or sensation. The person may experience the inability to walk, complete loss of movement in an arm or leg, blindness or deafness, or the absence or severe distortion of sensation over a portion of the body. This type of conversion typically appears in individuals of limited psychological sophistication and educational background. (Interestingly, these demographics represent

TABLE 9.3 Types of Conversion Reactions

Loss of function

Pseudoseizure

Pain reaction

a striking change from the turn of the century, when Freud and other investigators described conversion hysteria occurring among a sophisticated,
well-educated clientele.)

When evaluated neurologically, the conversion deficit is found to be only
a rough approximation of what would be expected based on neuroanatomi-
cal relationships. The person may appear unable to move a leg, yet when
the examiner draws attention to some other area, the leg inadvertently
moves. A disturbance in sensation may not conscribe to the anatomical
distribution of nerves, so that, for example, the person fails to register the
sensation of a pinprick over a square or circular patch on the body even
though the nerves are not distributed in that pattern. *In the absence of
neurological inconsistencies, conversion disorder is questionable as a
diagnosis.*

> A young man—previously an acrobat and dancer in the circus—enlisted in
> the Army during peacetime. He quickly found his new lifestyle monotonous
> compared to his traveling life with the circus. The discipline of military life was
> a rude awakening. He considered desertion but could not muster the courage.
> Without warning, he abruptly became unable to walk and could not feel
> anything in his legs. There was no previous history of this problem. In the face
> of this catastrophic event, he appeared relatively unconcerned. He was hospi-
> talized and officially discharged from the army shortly thereafter on a sur-
> geon's certificate of disability.
> The man's symptoms were never reconciled with any organic deficit. Grad-
> ually he regained function in his legs along with a return of normal sensation.
> Within a few months he left the hospital fully recovered. His diagnosis was
> conversion reaction. (Kolb, 1977)

Pseudoseizure (hystero-epilepsy) is a second type of conversion disorder,
occurring in a similar population. The person collapses on the floor or begins to experience thrashing or jerking movements. Inevitably the episode is
quite dramatic and hardly ever transpires in the absence of other people.

In many of these cases even a passing familiarity with organic seizures
will lead the observer to suspect a nonorganic origin. For example, the person, while appearing to have a grand mal seizure, may show obvious signs

of consciousness, such as speaking in a faint voice or responding to verbal command. The clinician should not forget, however, that certain seizures (complex partial) manifest as unusual forms of behavior. *All shifts in consciousness or behavior that recur in episodic fashion must be evaluated neurologically.* The clinician should be especially suspect of cases labeled conversion disorder that include a history of loss of bladder control, self-injury, or occurrence in the absence of other people. While frequently found in organic epilepsy cases, these findings are uncharacteristic of conversion. (The reader will recall that in the previous case of multiple sclerosis thought to be hysterical, the man had injured himself in two minor automobile accidents while driving alone. This was compelling evidence against a diagnosis of conversion disorder.)

Conversion reactions involving a *specific complaint* of pain—the third type—are particularly difficult to evaluate. As a general rule, nonmedical professionals should insist that persistent pain symptoms be evaluated by a physician. Medical specialists have at their disposal sophisticated testing procedures for differentiating organic from psychogenic pain. This is not a legitimate area of assessment for the nonspecialist. Even when an organic basis is not found initially, if pain persists or recurs, it should be reevaluated. Pain is an elusive phenomenon, one whose organic basis sometimes remains unidentified for long periods, despite intensive investigation.

Invariably, conversion disorder, regardless of type, is associated with significant interpersonal conflict. In fact, the symptom often provides at least a partial resolution. The resolution may be symbolic: A long-suffering woman confronted again and again with her husband's unfaithfulness suddenly becomes paralyzed in her right hand, rendering her unable to pull the trigger of the gun she has fantasized as the lethal weapon. Sometimes the conversion resolution to the conflict is more literal: a man confronted by the desire to tell off his tyrannical boss (but realistically unable to do so) becomes mute, thereby—in actuality as well as symbolically—resolving his conflict.

In addition to resolving conflict, psychiatric symptoms may produce secondary gain; that is, the person derives an additional advantage of personal attention from having become "ill." The role of "medical patient" affords a person certain privileges not otherwise available and sometimes tips the interpersonal balance in favor of the patient.

Finally, it is unusual for a person to have a single episode of conversion reaction. Unless it happens to be the initial occurrence, a previous history of unexplained somatic symptoms is characteristic. In the absence of a history of similar episodes, the clinician should be skeptical even when an initial neurological evaluation fails to turn up an organic cause. Similarly, the clinician should seriously question a diagnosis of conversion disorder that does not include the essential characteristics outlined in Table 9.4.

TABLE 9.4 Essential Characteristics of Conversion Reactions

Has no obvious organic basis

Occurs with sudden, dramatic onset in the midst of interpersonal conflict or other high-stress situation

Manifests as a single, prominent, physical symptom

> When she returned home from church, a 16-year-old girl complained of a severe headache and nausea. Shortly after going to the bathroom to take her medication (Fiorinal®), she was discovered by her parents, unconscious, lying on the floor. She was rushed to a nearby hospital, where in a few hours she regained consciousness. A neurologist declared she had suffered a conversion reaction. (LaWall & Ooomen, 1978)

At this juncture, even when rendered by a neurologist, the diagnosis of conversion reaction was inappropriate. The fact that the patient lost consciousness (in the absence of anyone else) combined with the absence of significant interpersonal stress or a previous history of similar episodes, constituted strong evidence against the diagnosis of conversion; nevertheless, the patient was admitted to a psychiatric hospital.

> The girl gave a two-year history of headaches. No neurological basis had been established. She had been followed by a physician and treated with Fiorinal, from which she obtained partial relief. Her headaches were one-sided. Often they were associated with nausea, blurred vision, and unsteadiness. Her friends said that during these headaches she walked as though she were intoxicated.
>
> The hospital staff described the patient as attractive and intelligent, depressed at times, but genuinely concerned about her condition. She talked openly with her psychologist about competing with her sister and described how good it felt to receive the special attention that she got from her mother when her headaches first started. Her MMPI showed a "conversion V" (allegedly seen in persons prone to conversion reactions). Based on her behavior on the unit, members of the nursing staff consistently described her, however, as a "healthy, normal teenager."
>
> Further neurological evaluation led to a diagnosis of "migraine headaches, basilar type."

Basilar migraine—a somewhat unusual variant of migraine—is characterized by a "sick" headache, usually only on one side, with unsteadiness and visual disturbances. It is primarily seen in adolescents, particularly girls.

This case illustrates the need to resist the diagnosis of conversion unless the evidence includes the essential characteristics I have noted. Although no organic basis had been found, other findings strongly argued against conversion disorder. She had multiple symptoms including headache, nausea, blurred vision, and unsteadiness. Furthermore, no escalation in the conflict with her sister or other stressful situation could be identified that would account for the present reaction. Another factor arguing against conversion was the patient's psychological awareness.

The diagnostic difficulties encountered in dealing with the symptom of pain are considerable. In a study of 250 patients with protracted head pain (after repeated negative medical consultations), 25% had an organic brain disorder accounting for their symptom (Friedman & Frazier, 1973). The clinician should always be uneasy categorizing pain as a conversion symptom.

In this chapter I have considered three forms of somatization, with the objective of familiarizing the reader with their clinical patterns, including their essential characteristics. The clinician should concentrate on recognizing inconsistencies that argue against somatization. As demonstrated in the various case histories, failure to detect organic disease, alone, is a fragile basis on which to conclude the presence of somatization. The casual application of terms like psychosomatic or hysterical is to be avoided.

REFERENCES

American Psychiatric Association (1987). *Diagnostic and statistical manual of mental disorders*. (Third Edition Revised), Washington, DC: American Psychiatric Association.

Cowley, D., & Roy-Byrne, P. (1987). Hyperventilation and panic disorder. *American Journal of Medicine, 83*, 929–937.

Dietch, J. (1984). Cerebral tumor presenting with panic attacks. *Psychosomatics, 25*, 861–863.

Dubousky, S. & Weissberg, M. (1978). *Clinical psychiatry in primary care*. Baltimore: Williams & Wilkins Co.

Feinglass, E., Arnett, F., Porsch, C., Zizic, T., & Steverns, M. (1976). Neuropsychiatric manifestations of systemic lupus erythematosus: diagnosis, clinical spectrum and relationship to other features of the disease. *Medicine, 55*, 323–339.

Friedman, A., & Frazier, S. (1973). Critique of the psychiatric treatment of chronic headache patients, in *Proceedings of the 5th World Congress of Psychiatrists*. New York: American Elsevier.

Fuller, D., M.D., Professor of Psychiatry, University of Texas at San Antonio Medical School. Personal communications, 1976.

Hellinger, W., Smith, T., Van Scoy, R., Spitzer, P., Fougacs, P., & Edson, R. (1988). Chronic fatigue syndrome and the diagnostic utility of antibody to Epstein-Barr early antigen. *Journal of the American Medical Association, 260*, 971–973.

Joffe, R., Rubinow, D., Denicoff, K., Maher, M., & Sindelar, W. (1986). Depression and carcinoma of the pancreas. *General Hospital Psychiatry, 8*, 241–245.

Kaminsky, M., & Slavney, P. (1976). Methodology and personality in Briquet's syndrome: a reappraisal. *American Journal of Psychiatry, 133*, 58–88.

Kellner, R. (1987). Hypochondriasis and somatization. *Journal of the American Medical Association, 258*, 2718–2722.

Kirmayer, L., Robbins, J., & Kapusta, M. (1988). Somatization and depression in fibromyalgia syndrome. *American Journal of Psychiatry, 145*, 950–954.

Klerman, G. (1988). Overview of the cross-national collaborative panic study. *Archives of General Psychiatry, 45*, 407–412.

Kolb, L. (1977) *Modern clinical psychiatry.* Philadelphia: W. B. Saunders Co.

LaWall, J., & Ooommen, K. (1978). Basilar artery migraine presenting as conversion hysteria. *Journal of Nervous and Mental Disease, 166*, 809–811.

Martin, J. (1979). Physical disease manifesting as psychiatric disorders. In G. Usdin & J. Lewis (eds.). *Psychiatry in General Medical Practice* (337–351). New York: McGraw-Hill.

Mukerjiv, V., & Alpert, M. (1987). Panic disorder: a frequent occurrrence in patients with chest pain and normal coronary arteries. *Angiology, 38*, 236–240.

Pincus, J., & Tucker, G. (1974). *Behavioral neurology.* New York: Oxford University Press.

Woodruff, R., Goodwin, D., & Guse, S. (1974). *Psychiatric diagnosis.* New York: Oxford University Press.

Yaskin, J. (1931). Nervous symptoms as earliest manifestations of carcinoma of the pancreas. *JAMA, 96*, 1664–1668.

Chapter 10

The Old and the Young

They say an old man is twice a child.   —William Shakespeare

The basic principles we have considered for identifying psychological masquerade are generally applicable regardless of a patient's age. In this chapter we will take a special look at psychological masquerades that occur in children and in older persons.

AGING AND ORGANIC MENTAL DISORDERS

Reaching old age is becoming commonplace, and older persons are at increased risk for diseases that frequently cause psychological masquerade.

A key concept to keep in mind regarding older people is this: *Mental deterioration is not synonymous with aging.* It's essential to avoid the trap of assuming that notable mental decline goes hand in hand with getting older. It's simply not true. One author has recommended "prophylactic injections against the notion that old age involves imbecility" (Comfort, 1980). The fact that an individual is aged should not be accepted automatically as an explanation for mental and emotional decline.

Old age is not the cause of senility!

Furthermore, not all senility is the same. Some forms are caused by correctable conditions. They are not expressions of true dementia; they only mimic it. This is one of the reasons why properly identifying psychological masquerade in the elderly is so very important. Other forms of senility, unfortunately, are not reversible, although with the tremendous strides being made in the neurosciences, this may change in the near future.

IRREVERSIBLE DEMENTIAS

Approximately 10% of persons 65 years or older have senile dementia (Fox, Topel, & Huckman, 1975). Several diseases produce this clinical picture which resembles what I described earlier as slow-onset brain syndrome (SOBS).

Alzheimer's Disease

Several million Americans 65 years or older have Alzheimer's disease. Research findings suggest that this condition (involving widespread progressive destruction of brain cells), is identical to presenile dementia which strikes persons in mid-life. Alzheimer's disease—the etiology of which is unknown—accounts for approximately 50% of all cases of dementia (Comfort, 1980). It virtually always presents as failing memory and disorientation. When they first appear, these deficits can be so subtle that only in retrospect are they recognized as signaling the onset of dementia. Relentlessly, the deficits become more obvious. Appointments may be forgotten, stories repeated, mistakes made. The person may lose his way in his own neighborhood. There may be transient periods of depression and anxiety. The person is less spontaneous. Facial expression becomes unchanging, vacant in appearance. Activities and people that in the past were important become of little interest. Apathy settles in, only to be interrupted periodically by unexplained moments of panic or hyperexcitability.

As Alzheimer's disease progresses, difficulty reading and solving simple problems and calculations is encountered. Finding the right word becomes problematic. Sound judgment is lost. Movement becomes impaired, characterized by unsteadiness and a shortened gait. In some cases, seizures occur. Later, bowel and bladder control may be lost.

Early in the evolution of Alzheimer's disease, it can be mistaken for reactive depression. As it progresses, however, the evidence for organicity builds; in later stages it is readily identifiable as a neurological condition.

Multiple Infarct Dementia

Multiple infarct dementia is associated with arteriosclerotic changes in blood vessels. These changes increase the risk of blockage and the death of small areas of the brain supplied by the affected vessel. (The term *infarct* refers to dead tissue produced by arterial insufficiency.) Usually, persons who develop multiinfarct dementia suffer from high blood pressure.

This form of irreversible dementia accounts for roughly 15% of cases of dementia; another 20% of cases occur in conjunction with Alzheimer's disease. The clinical symptoms accompanying these two conditions are virtually indistinguishable but have somewhat different courses. Whereas Alzheimer's disease proceeds as a gradual deterioration, multiple infarct dementia progresses in stepwise fashion, usually punctuated by dramatic episodes of mental decline. Clinical detection hinges on the identification of core features of brain syndrome that may be overshadowed by psychological symptoms such as depression and anxiety related to declining cognitive ability and the threat of losing control.

Treatment for both of these forms of dementia is limited, but practical counseling can be extremely helpful; thus, early recognition is important to the patient and his or her family. If these irreversible dementias are correctly identified rather than being mistaken for crazy behavior or "getting old," families can be educated as to how best to cope with future problems.

REVERSIBLE DEMENTIAS

Approximately one out of every ten cases of persons with symptoms suggestive of senile dementia have a potentially correctable organic disorder (Cummings, Benson, & LoVerne, 1980).

Medication Intoxications

The most common form of reversible dementia results from medication and drug intoxications. Older persons consume more than their share of both prescription and over-the-counter medications, to which they are supersensitive. Small amounts can cause major problems.

As a general rule, the older people are, the more sensitive they are to drugs. Those over the age of 80 are twice as sensitive as persons under age 60 (Hurtwitz, 1969). Even a drug as seemingly innocuous as acetaminophen (Tylenol®) can produce adverse effects such as confusion and hallucinations. Given the sudden onset of mental or emotional disturbances in an elderly person, drugs should immediately go to the top of the list of possible causes.

Dosages of medication well tolerated by younger persons routinely cause adverse reactions in the elderly, primarily because many drugs—especially psychoactive drugs—remain in the elderly body longer, exerting stronger and more prolonged effects. Several factors contribute to this delayed metabolism of drugs. First of all, due to an age-related decline in cardiac proficiency, circulation time lengthens in older people, so that it takes longer for a drug to pass through the body's drug "breakdown stations," namely the kidneys and liver. Also, these organs themselves undergo aging changes that render them less efficient. The kidneys become less effective filters, and the liver produces less of the enzymes essential for drug metabolism. A final factor relates to the relative increase in body fat that goes along with getting older. This makes for a prolonged response to psychoactive drugs because most of these substances are stored in the body's fat reserves. From these storage depots, medications are slowly released similar to the pattern seen with time-release capsules.

> A twice-widowed man in his mid-eighties, known to his friends and family for his aggressive pursuit of living, became apathetic and withdrawn. He would sit in a chair most of the day, showing little concern for food, friends, or any other of his previous interests. Earlier, on several occasions, he had parked his car and then forgotten where it was. When for the third time he reported it stolen, the police threatened to revoke his license.
>
> His local doctor thought the problem was old age, but the man was referred for more extensive evaluation. He was coherent but exhibited a degree of confusion. No evidence for infections or other commonly encountered physical diseases was discovered.
>
> Although initially the man denied using any drugs, further inquiry showed that after the death of his first wife (many years before) he had started taking a butabarbital tablet nightly in order to sleep. When, following the death of his second wife, his sleeplessness returned, he was prescribed a second sedative (Quaalude). His problems related to taking the two medications together.
>
> Despite strong protests from the old man, the sleeping medications were discontinued. Within 10 days his zest for activity had reappeared, his appetite had returned, and his confusion had cleared. He started socializing again and had no further incidents of misplacing his car. (Comfort, 1980)

Certain medications are frequent perpetrators of psychological masquerade among the elderly, in part because of their widespread use. Anti-inflammatory drugs often cause depression; more rarely, psychosis. Many of the diuretics, due to their potassium-depleting effect, produce fatigue, apathy, and depression. Older persons can easily be overloaded with antianxiety medications and sedatives. Many of these drugs have prolonged action times, setting the stage for significant buildup over a few days with resulting drowsiness and listlessness. This problem is largely avoided by using drugs which have no active metabolites such as the benzodiazepine, oxazepam (Serax®).

Cimetidine (Tagemet®) is widely prescribed for stomach hyperacidity, dyspepsia, and ulcers. Even small amounts have caused delirium and psychosis in older persons.

Older persons are often given small doses of neuroleptic medication for agitation. What often goes unattended is the rapid development of drug-induced parkinsonism. The person becomes stiff and unable to move normally. Stooped posture, a halting slow gait, and drooling appear. Spontaneity and normal facial expressions are lost. Upon cessation of the drug, these complications quickly disappear.

Digitalis (and its various derivatives) has been a cornerstone medication in the management of heart failure; and, even though in recent times it has been replaced to some extent by newer preparations, this venerable remedy is still widely used, particularly among the elderly. The problem with digitalis is that the dose required for a therapeutic response is close to the amount that proves to be toxic. Even when serum levels of digitalis are within the therapeutic range, various mental and emotional aberrations can occur. One report described two men being treated with digoxin (digitalis derivative), both in their 70s, who despite "nontoxic" levels of digoxin, became extremely tearful. When the medication was reduced the tearfulness disappeared (Eisendrath & Sweeney, 1987).

Older persons, as noted earlier, are especially vulnerable to anticholinergic agents. The therapeutic benefits are often outweighed by adverse effects.

> A 74-year-old man with tremulous movements and body rigidity was diagnosed as having Parkinson's disease. Despite treatment with antiparkinsonian medications, over the next two years his memory deteriorated and he began to have difficulty finding the right words to express himself. He became disoriented and developed paranoid delusions and hallucinations. He fell into a severe depression with uncontrollable crying spells.
>
> After two years he was referred to a special clinic for Parkinson's disease. The preliminary impression was that he was now suffering additionally from "cortical dementia, probably Alzheimer's type." Neuropsychological testing, however, suggested drug intoxication. Consequently, the patient's anticholinergic medication was tapered off over the next eight days. One week later there had been a dramatic improvement in the patient's memory and mood. His wife described him as a "new man." (Kurlan & Como, 1988)

For the elderly, there are no "minor" tranquilizers! The medications they take often put them at risk for mental dysfunction.

Subdural Hematoma

A subdural hematoma is a collection of blood in the space just under the dura, the outermost covering of the brain. The most common cause is traumatic injury to the head that tears the small veins traversing the subdural space. Symptoms, (which can be primarily mental or behavioral), stem from increased intracranial pressure and encroachment of the developing blood clot on surrounding brain tissue.

Accidental falls among older people place them at special risk for subdurals. This risk is further increased if the elderly person also has a problem with alcohol. Given a history of abrupt mental deterioration or significant behavioral change in an older person, the clinician should always inquire about accidents or falls. The possibility should not be completely dismissed, simply because there is no recall of a fall or a blow to the head. In a study of 75 cases of subdural hematoma, one out of three lacked any known history of head trauma. (Stuteville & Welch, 1958) Sometimes bruising about the head or eyes will suggest the possibility of head trauma, even when the person cannot recall the injury. The clinician should be on the alert for such tell-tale signs.

In contrast to acute subdural hematomas, the chronic variety evolves more slowly and is more subtle in its clinical presentation. Chronic subdurals become symptomatic over a period of days to weeks. Symptoms are varied, but may include inattentiveness, social withdrawal, disinterest, and intellectual decline. Psychotic manifestations are also possible. Headache is a frequent finding and it may be intermittent. Neurological deficits such as weakness in the arms, legs, or muscles of the face sometimes readily indicate the organic nature of this condition. Such signs, however, are not invariably present.

An elderly man, active and in good health, had occupied himself with gardening and odd-jobbing for his neighbors. Just prior to Christmas, while digging under an apple tree, he struck his head sharply on a low-hanging branch. He felt dazed but quickly recovered without losing consciousness. The following day, walking home from a neighbor's house, he inexplicably fell over in the road. He quickly got to his feet and walked on, but an observer noticed that he seemed to be walking oddly.

Over the next few days, the man inexplicably became disorganized, excessively sleepy, and "completely unlike his former self." He also lost control of his bladder.

Three weeks later he was admitted to a hospital, where he was found to have right-sided facial weakness. Arteriography showed a large subdural hematoma. It was evacuated surgically. The man had an excellent recovery and experienced no residual problems. (Pygott & Street, 1950)

The treatment outcomes for chronic subdural hematomas are gratifying. One study of 52 elderly patients showed that 75% were restored to their prior level of functioning following surgery. (Raskind & Glover, 1972)

Normal Pressure Hydrocephalus

Another masquerade to watch for in the elderly is normal pressure hydrocephalus. This condition results from an overabundance of cerebral spinal fluid. It usually affects persons in their sixties and seventies. Although several diseases can produce this problem, most cases have no obvious cause; even so, this type of hydrocephalus often can be corrected surgically by implanting a shunt to drain off excessive fluid.

Psychiatric symptoms, particularly apathy, may be the first sign of normal pressure hydrocephalus. As the condition progresses, forgetfulness and day-to-day shifts in the ability to think emerge along with a peculiar deficit in walking. This so-called *magnetic gait* results from difficulty initiating each step. It is as though the person's feet are stuck to the floor. The person adapts by widening his stance and taking slow, short steps. The third classic symptom is loss of bladder control.

When cognitive decline is associated with difficulty walking and urinary incontinence, normal pressure hydrocephalus should go to the top of the lists of suspects.

If detected early, normal pressure hydrocephalus can be successfully treated. The earlier the diagnosis, the more favorable the outcome.

A 58-year-old man became delusional, insisting the he had given his wife a strange illness. He also believed that people in his home town were talking about him and meant to do him harm. When he was finally admitted to a hospital, it was established that he had been suffering from depression for the past eight months. He had had difficulty remembering things and was unable to concentrate for even the shortest time. His walking was awkward and unsteady.

A series of neurological studies (including an EEG, brain scan, and skull X rays) were judged to be normal. Together, a neurologist and psychiatrist concluded that there was no organic brain disease and diagnosed the problem as psychotic depression.

Over the next six months, the man was treated with haloperidol (antipsychotic) and imipramine (antidepressant). His symptoms showed some improvement.

A year later, however, he was readmitted after a recurrence of his symptoms and deterioration in his ability to walk. During this hospitalization, he was treated with electroconvulsive therapy (ECT) and discharged again.

Within two months he returned again, acutely agitated and paranoid, having impulsively attempted suicide with pills. He evidenced a striking memory deficit as well as impairment in his ability to think abstractly. Specialized studies produced findings consistent with a diagnosis of normal pressure hydrocephalus. A year later, after a surgical shunting procedure, he was 80–90% his normal self. (Price & Tucker, 1977)

There have been reported cases of schizophrenic-like illness in association with the symptoms of normal pressure hydrocephalus. Allegedly, surgical shunting resulted in the amelioration of the "schizophrenia." (Lying-Tunnell, 1979). This is an intriguing finding, suggesting the possibility of a special hydrocephalic subcategory of schizophrenia.

Losing One's Senses

Older persons are prone to diminished sensory acuity. As hearing and vision decline, a person may become depressed. Paranoid thinking is another common reaction to sensory loss. Here, paranoia is a way of understanding (albeit irrationally), a chaotic world stemming from sensory gaps. *Paraphrenia* is a term applied to old-age paranoia that surfaces in the absence of a history of schizophrenia. Several studies have suggested that partial deafness plays an important causative role (Eisdorfer, 1980).

Failing sight can also precipitate psychiatric symptoms. Evidence for this comes from studies of elderly persons who undergo surgery for cataracts. Following surgery, it is imperative that a patient's eyes be covered with black patches. This state of iatrogenic blindness often leads to rapid-onset brain syndrome.

Another clinically misleading aspect of aging is the decline in the body's ability to signal the presence of disease. For example, the characteristic manifestations of pneumonia—fever, chills, increased respiratory rate, and pain on breathing—may be quite muted or even absent in an elderly person. Instead, the person may simply become lethargic and incoherent.

This absence or softening of symptoms can mask such serious physical disorders as heart attack, heart failure, and pulmonary insufficiency. Whereas in a younger person these conditions are readily identifiable as medical problems, among the elderly only the psychological and behavioral changes due to secondary brain failure may be observable. This is why a clinician should pursue even the most innocuous appearing physical complaints in an older person.

A 75-year-old widow had been living alone. Although she was said to have somewhat eccentric religious beliefs, she had never before exhibited psychotic behavior; never, that is, until she abruptly expressed religious delusions and became suspicious and agitated. After being found setting her house on fire because of "instructions from Jesus Christ," she was admitted to a psychiatric unit.

Her heart rate was quite rapid (160 beats per minute). An EKG showed supraventricular tachycardia that was causing heart failure. After 3 days of treatment with digoxin (a drug used for certain irregularities in heart rhythm as well as heart failure) her rate had slowed to 86 beats per minute, and her symptoms of heart failure were improving. Simultaneously, she had become much more lucid. By the following week her acute psychosis had disappeared, leaving in its place an aging woman with a slightly eccentric personality. (Clark, 1970)

Temporal Arteritis

Temporal arteritis is a chronic inflammatory condition primarily of the arteries supplying the head. It is rarely seen in persons before the age of 60; typically, patients are in their 70s and 80s. The earliest manifestations include malaise, muscle aches and pains, abdominal discomfort, weight loss, depression, and a sore tongue. Eventually, the patient complains of severe headaches localized to the temporal arteries on the side of the head. Usually, the arteries will be swollen and exquisitely painful to touch.

The problem for the clinician is that restlessness, insomnia, disorientation, severe depression, or frank psychosis can mask the true nature of temporal arteritis. Proper recognition depends on noting the characteristic temporal headache pattern in conjunction with psychiatric symptoms in an older person.

Vitamin B$_{12}$ Deficiency (Pernicious Anemia)

Vitamin B$_{12}$ deficiency is found in roughly 3–10% of patients over age 65 (Carethers, 1988). The most common cause is related to failure of the lining of the stomach to produce a substance known as intrinsic factor. (Understandably, B$_{12}$ deficiency sometimes occurs in persons who have undergone partial or full removal of the stomach.) Vitamin B$_{12}$ is stored in the liver. When it is no longer being produced in the stomach, the reserves are gradually depleted, thus accounting for the insidious onset of symptoms. Sometimes this disease is nutritional in origin. Strict vegetarians or elderly persons living on "tea and toast" are particularly susceptible.

Eventually, persons with B$_{12}$ deficiency show obvious neurological deficits such as numbness and tingling in their fingers and toes and severe imbalance when walking. Blood testing reveals a characteristic anemia. Psychiatric changes, however, can occur first, giving rise to psychological masquerade.

Pseudodementia

What looks like dementia is not always the real thing.

Pseudodementia is a different kind of masquerade that occurs among the elderly. In essence it is depression masquerading as dementia. It is critically important to avoid mislabeling a patient as having Alzheimer's disease, particularly if they are suffering from a readily treatable condition such as depression. It is estimated that 10–20% of depressed elderly patients have substantial cognitive deficits—confusion, memory loss, diminished problem-solving—easily mistaken for dementia. To further complicate the clinician's task, a sizable number of Alzheimer dementia patients become severely depressed. There are several important differentiating points (Reynolds et al., 1988; Wells, 1979).

Pseudodementia tends to evolve rapidly in contrast to the more gradual onset of most cases of dementia. Furthermore, whereas the depressed (pseudodemented) patient frequently complains of losing his mind or being unable to think, the person with Alzheimer's disease works hard to cover up the problem, bringing as little attention as possible to his deficit. This includes efforts to mislead others, including the clinician. The truly demented patient will make significant if not outlandish mistakes. The pseudodemented patient, in contrast, will respond frequently with "I don't know" answers or near misses.

Table 10.1 provides a list of causes of reversible dementias.

CHILDREN AND ORGANIC MENTAL DISORDERS

As a general rule, any noteable psychological symptom in a child, when occurring for the first time or when associated with physical illness, should be thoroughly medically evaluated. In the absence of significant stress or a specific precipitating event, mental aberrations in children are more likely organic than psychological.

Declining School Performance

School performance is a sensitive indicator of the well-being of a child. With the exception of reactive depression (which is usually readily apparent), a

TABLE 10.1 Causes of Reversible Dementia

Intracranial Conditions	**Drugs (continued)**
Meningiomas	Benzodiazapines
Subdural hematomas	Barbiturates
Hydrocephalus	Clonidine
Epilepsy	Methyldopa
Multiple sclerosis	Propranolol hydrochloride
Wilson's disease	Atropine and related compounds
Systemic Illnesses	**Heavy Metals**
Pulmonary insufficiency	Mercury
Cardiac arrhythmia	Arsenic
Severe anemia	Lead
Polycythemia vera	Thallium
Uremia	**Exogenous Toxins and**
Hyponatremia	**Industrial Agents**
Hepatic encephalopathy	Trichloroethylene
Porphyria	Toluene
Hyperlipidemia	Carbon disulfide
Deficiency States	Organophosphates
B_{12} deficiency	Carbon monoxide
Pellegra	Alcohol
Folate deficiency	**Infections**
Endocrinopathies	General paresis
Addison's disease	Chronic meningitis
Myxedema	Cerebral abscess
Hypoparathyroidism	Cysticercosis
Hyperparathyroidism	Whipple's disease
Recurrent hypoglycemia	Progressive multifocal
Cushing's disease	leukoencephalopathy
Hyperthyroidism	Encephalitis
Drugs	**Collagen-Vascular and Vascular**
Disulfiram	**Disorders**
Lithium carbonate	Systemic lupus erythematosus
Phenothiazines	Temporal arteritis
Phenytoin	Sarcoidosis

Adopted from Cummings, Benson, and LoVerne, 1980. Reversible dementia. *JAMA, 243.*

substantial decline in a child's school performance is most often a reflection of organic dysfunction. In one report of children with neurological disease—all of whom had initially received psychiatric diagnoses—declining school performance had shown up early in the course of the disorder in every case (Mark & Gath, 1978). Explaining declining school performance in terms of family dynamics without a neurological evaluation is risky business.

A 12-year-old Yugoslavian-born child was brought up in Iceland by his aunt until his parents, who had emigrated to the United States several years earlier, called for him. Although the boy initially had some difficulty with the language, for six months he progressed well in school. Then, mysteriously, his school performance rapidly declined.

At first this was attributed to cultural shock. Counseling was started along with psychotropic medications; but the boy's academic performance continued to deteriorate.

Another six months passed before a neurological consultation was sought. Based on EEG and spinal fluid findings (along with the clinical observation of spastic movements), a diagnosis of subacute sclerosing panencephalitis was made, for which, unfortunately, there is no known cure.

Over the next three years, the child became severely demented and suffered frequent seizures before eventually succumbing to this tragic condition. (Laufer & Taranth, 1979)

The outcome of this slow virus infection is always fatal. In this case its initial clinical manifestation was a dramatic decline in school performance.

Psychosis in Children

Before the age of 12, psychotic symptoms are relatively rare. When a child has hallucinations or delusions or relates in a grossly inappropriate manner, organic mental disorder is the most likely explanation.

Autism is a form of organic psychosis occurring in early childhood (Ornitz & Ritvo, 1976). Although the precise neurological deficit has yet to be firmly established, the fact that autism appears virtually from birth, that it is characterized by highly stereotypical behavior changes, exhibits significant genetic loading, and is associated with neurobiologic abnormalities (as reflected in electroencephalograms and CT scans) provides persuasive evidence for an organic basis (Volkmar & Cohen, 1988).

Autistic children exhibit abnormalities that fall into four categories: severe speech disruption, peculiar responses to stimulation, disturbed relatedness, and disturbances of motion.

Autistic children fail to acquire meaningful speech, either remaining mute or producing weird, high-pitched sounds having no recognizable meaning. In those few instances where speech does appear, usually it is late in onset and has notable peculiarities. The child may repeat phrases over and over again in echo-like fashion (echolalia). Usually, there is an absence of normal rhythm and tone and a highly mechanical quality to what limited speech exists.

Autistic children respond inappropriately to their immediate environment. For example, there may be no observable reaction to sounds or normally compelling sights. Periods of intense staring from which nothing can distract the child are typical. It is as though an invisible barrier is raised between the outside world and the child. As if to overcome this insulation, the child resorts to strange, self-stimulating activities, such as endless whirling, rocking, or head-rolling.

Typically, physical contact with other persons is shunned. There is a decided preference for constancy which is upset by the presence of other people. Not surprisingly, normal social skills fail to evolve, including even the ability to smile.

The autistic child exhibits strange movements. For example, he may walk on his toes for extended periods. Body-rocking, characterized by swaying to and fro, is also common, as is a peculiar hand flapping in front of the child's own face. At times these aberrations are replaced by extended periods of "frozen" postures.

Autism usually is fully manifest by the age of 3. Treatment is limited, but proper diagnosis helps to avoid inappropriate therapy and unwarranted parental guilt. Furthermore, once it is recognized that the child's autistic problem is not psychological, a more realistic management program can be instituted.

A host of other organic conditions, including brain tumors, central nervous system infections, and drug intoxications cause childhood psychosis. The important point to remember is that psychotic symptoms in children should never be interpreted in psychological terms without first carefully evaluating for an organic mental disorder.

Childhood Seizures

As with seizures in adults, if gross motor movements occur during a child's seizures, usually there is no difficulty recognizing the problem as neurological. There are childhood seizure disorders, however, that manifest predominantly as behavioral changes. The symptoms seen in temporal lobe epilepsy are similar to those described for adults in Chapter 7. This disorder should always be suspected in children experiencing unexplained shifts in consciousness, especially when combined with semipurposeful movements and a preceding aura.

Petit mal epilepsy occurs *predominantly* in children. It is marked by sudden, brief lapses in consciousness, during which the child momentarily stops what he is doing. If an episode comes on while the child is talking, he stops in mid-sentence. If the period of "absence" is quite brief, the child may resume talking where he has left off. With longer attacks, a degree of confusion or bewilderment usually persists after consciousness returns.

When attacks of petit mal epilepsy follow one another in rapid-fire fashion (so that the child never quite recovers from one before being overcome by the next), the condition is called "status," an allusion to its sustained nature. It is not difficult to envision how a child experiencing status petit mal becomes disoriented and acts in a highly peculiar fashion.

Although most attacks of petit mal arise spontaneously, sometimes they have specific precipitants. Music, light, even reading and emotional stress have been known to trigger seizures in predisposed children. Some cases result in sudden collapse, where the child for no apparent reasons falls to the ground or floor. Due to their dramatic nature, these seizures are sometimes misconstrued as hysterical or feigned.

> For several years, a 9-year-old girl had frequently passed out just as she was leaving home for school. Although at first extremely concerned, her parents eventually decided she was faking. Her family physician concluded that she was suffering from a school phobia.
>
> After several years, the child was referred for a complete neurological examination. A detailed history disclosed that these episodes happened only on bright, sunny days. With the aid of a series of EEG studies, it was found that exposure to bright light did indeed precipitate these seizures. Each morning when the child stepped out her front door into a bright morning sun, she lost consciousness and fell to the ground. (Livingston, Pauli, & Bruce, 1980)

Psychiatric Symptoms and Disorders of Movement

The unexpected association between psychiatric symptoms and abnormal movements previously discussed with reference to adult disorders, is also found in certain childhood conditions.

Wilson's disease results from a genetic abnormality affecting the transport of copper within the body. This causes a destructive "plating-out" onto body tissues, mainly the liver and brain.

Approximately 20% of these cases initially manifest *solely* as anxiety, depression, mania, or paranoid thinking. In other cases psychiatric symptoms are seen in conjunction with strange movements—tremors, jerkiness, or subtle twisting of the extremities. Sometimes, symptoms of hepatitis, stemming from living damage, will also be present.

As Wilson's disease progresses, the child's facial expression becomes vacant; control of emotional expression is increasingly tenuous, giving rise to inappropriate crying and laughing. Full-blown psychotic symptoms are not uncommon.

For two years school officials had described the child as "emotionally disturbed." In addition, she showed a noticeable lack of coordination in physical education activities. Finally, when her emotional problems persisted, she was sent to a children's psychiatric unit, and treated for childhood schizophrenia. The increasing severity of her jerky movements, however, finally led to a suspicion of neurological disease. A slit-lamp eye examination showed the characteristic "golden ring" in the cornea of her eyes. Laboratory tests confirmed the diagnosis of Wilson's disease.

Unfortunately, by this time the condition was far advanced. Despite the use of a chelating agent (for the elimination of excessive body copper), the child continued to deteriorate. She expired one month after her condition had been diagnosed. (Malamud, 1975)

Early detection of Wilson's disease is crucial; otherwise the patient is condemned to a premature death.

Tourette's syndrome (TS) was first reported in 1885 by the French neurologist after whom it was named, Gilles de la Tourette. It is an uncanny disorder that in its most severe form makes a person appear possessed. Nervous tics and strange, jerky movements are combined with compulsive behaviors, including involuntary utterances, varying from indecipherable growls to explosive outbursts of explicit, dirty words.

Typically, TS has its onset in childhood. It may begin with excessive eye-blinking, followed by facial tics and grimacing. With time these involuntary movements are joined by compulsive behaviors. The child may be compelled to touch or smell things or to repeat commonplace activities such as squatting, hopping, or jumping. Later (in roughly 50% of TS patients), uncontrolled utterances appear that initially may be mistaken for coughing or throat clearing. They go on to become unmistakable verbalizations of dirty words (coprolalia). The TS patient struggles against this compulsion. He may cover his mouth or run from the situation, but when he is unsuccessful, the result is an embarrassing flood of graphic expletives ("fuck, shit, cock . . .").

Research on TS suggests an excessive amount of brain dopamine. This could account for the favorable response to haloperidol (and other dopamine blocking agents) experienced by a majority of patients. Treatment, however, is by no means without its drawbacks. Some patients find themselves slowed down physically and mentally.

In his book, *The Man Who Mistook His Wife For A Hat,* Oliver Sacks describes a patient named Ray who had accommodated to his TS well enough to be a weekend jazz drummer of considerable local renown, famous for his wild musical improvisations. Although nine years of treatment with haloperidol dramatically changed his life for the better, his drum playing suffered. Finally, a compromise was worked out: Ray took his medication on weekdays, but discontinued it for his weekend jazz performances so he could "let fly" (Sacks, 1987).

Despite the attention given to the full-blown syndrome, most cases of TS are mild in severity. A study of 142,636 children enrolled in public and private school documented a prevalence of 27.7/100,000. Of the 41 identified cases, only three had an "impairing, diagnosable disorder." Most suffered only from tics and other minor changes in movement. Roughly half had obsessive–compulsive tendencies. Family histories of TS or tics were common (Caine, 1988).

Inappropriate referrals for traditional psychotherapy are frequently made for this neurological syndrome. One study found that the initial symptoms of TS were usually mistaken for signs of tension and nervousness (Golder, 1977).

Attention-deficit hyperactivity disorder (minimal brain dysfunction) applies to persons who have extremely short attention spans making concentration and normal social interaction impossible. This is the most common psychiatric disorder of children, estimated to occur in 4–10% of pre-adolescents. Understandably, it leads to poor school performance, erratic and impulsive behavior, and poor social relations. It has also been associated with increased risk for delinquent and criminal behavior.

Although hyperactivity is often associated with attention deficit disorder, this is not invariably the case (Edelbrock, Costello, & Kessler, 1984). When it is present, however, the child may be mistakenly labeled as anxious, impulsive, or incorrigible.

In the *Diagnostic and Statistical Manual of Mental Disorders, Revised* (DSM-III-R), 14 defining symptoms in three clusters are listed: inattention (5), impulsivity (6) and hyperactivity (3). According to the DSM-III-R criteria, 8 of these 14 symptoms are required for diagnosis. If criteria are present *without* hyperactivity, the condition is termed "undifferentiated attention-deficit disorder."

Surprisingly, recent evidence suggests that children who are inattentive and not hyperactive have more school difficulty, more unhappiness, and greater risk for long-term social and academic problems. The observation has also been made (contrary to previous belief) that attention deficit problems may *not* be more common among boys than girls; girls, however, are much more likely to go unrecognized in that they exhibit less hyperactivity and disruptive behavior (Berry, Shaywitz, & Shaywitz, 1985).

In screening for attention-deficit disorder, the clinician needs to confirm that the child cannot sustain normal attention for more than a few minutes *even while engaged in a rewarding or pleasurable activity.*

It is now clear that there is a biological predisposition to this condition; therefore, it is not too surprising to find that medication has been used effectively. Paradoxically, many children with attentional deficits respond favorably to stimulants such as methylphenidate (Ritalin®). Although this form of treatment sometimes has been applied too liberally, when given to children who meet strict criteria, the positive changes with respect to school and social performance are often dramatic. This in turn has beneficial consequences for the child's self-image.

Adjusting the dose of methylphenidate (or other stimulants) can be a delicate balancing act: not enough and the child's condition remains unimproved; too much and the problem of inattention becomes compounded by tremulousness, difficulty sleeping, and increasing fearfulness that may turn into full-fledged paranoia.

> A six-year-old boy lived with his mother and infant sister in a government-subsidized, high-rise apartment. His mother described him as always on the go and constantly getting into things. After an episode during which the child covered himself and the entire apartment with baby powder, he was taken to see a psychiatrist.
>
> The history (along with his interview evaluation) revealed that, despite normal hearing, the boy often failed to listen and had trouble complying with directions. Also, he typically failed to carry things to completion. At preschool he had been described by his teacher as distractable, defiant, and impulsive. He was involved in fights and often spoke out of turn.
>
> In the psychiatrist's office, despite being friendly and outgoing, he was difficult to interview because he was so distractible and hyperactive.
>
> He was given a diagnosis of attention-deficit disorder with hyperactivity and treated with methylphenidate. In a short while, however, his teacher complained that he was acting erratically. For long periods he would appear "spacy," looking like a "zombie." Abruptly, he would snap out of it only to go into a rage reaction. At other times he would cower in the corner of the classroom, looking extremely frightened and describing insects and spiders that no one else could see. Understandably, his academic performance plummeted.
>
> His mother took him to another clinic for a second opinion. The original diagnosis was confirmed, but he was thought to be having toxic side effects to the methylphenidate. The dosage was lowered. His erratic behavior disappeared and his schoolwork improved significantly, as did his personal relationships at home and at school. (Meller & Lyle, 1987)

It was originally thought that attention-deficit disorder occurred only in children; that it was a condition a person grew out of. It is now known that this is not invariably the case. The persistence of the problem into adulthood has been well described (Wender, 1987).

Sensory deficits, such as hearing and visual impairment, often cause behavioral disturbances in children. The inability to see or hear adequately can create considerable frustration in a child; but, because there is no basis for comparison, the child may never complain about these deficits. Hearing and vision should be routinely tested in children with psychiatric symptoms. The clinician can grossly screen for problems by having the child visualize an object or printed words on a wall across the room. Similarly, a soft whisper when the child is not looking, if not responded to, provides evidence of a hearing deficit. These simple screening procedures, however, should not supplant the use of standardized testing for vision and hearing when there is evidence that the child suffers from a sensory deficit.

Bulimia is on the rise. It affects women primarily, and commonly begins in late adolescence. Characteristically, there are secret episodes of binge eating over which the person feels little sense of control. In addition, self-induced vomiting, laxatives, or diuretics are used for weight control. Through all of this the person holds steadfastly to a distorted view of her actual weight.

I bring up the subject of bulimia because it can become complicated by serious medical problems of the patient's own making. The clinician should be alert to these medical complications. For example, some bulimics resort to syrup of ipecac as a means of inducing vomiting. Ipecac is a likely candidate, as it is effective, cheap, and available without a prescription. There's only one problem: ipecac is highly toxic to skeletal and cardiac muscle. As the person uses ipecac more and more, it works less well, resulting in greater absorption of the syrup itself until toxic levels are reached.

One report described a 19-year-old bulimic woman who used ipecac so extensively that she eventually could only walk in a waddling gait and could not hold her hands above her head for more than a few seconds, due to severe muscle weakness. She also suffered from dilation and weakness of the heart with resulting shortness of breath (Friedman, Seine, Roberts, & Fremouw, 1987).

Another complication of bulimia is the depletion of the body's stores of magnesium and potassium. Hypomagnesemia usually results from chronic diuretic and laxative use. Roughly a quarter of bulimic patients have this complication. Symptoms include restlessness, decreased concentration, and poor memory. Bulimics are also susceptible to potassium loss from the overuse of diuretics. Apathy, depression, and fatigue are common. If the potassium loss is too great, life-threatening cardiac arrhythmias may arise.

Twenty percent of bulimic women are chemically dependent and are susceptible to the adverse effects of the various drugs they use (Mickley, 1988). Diet pills (phenylpropanolamine), if used for prolonged periods, produce suspiciousness and may eventually lead to paranoid psychosis.

In short, an initial problem of bulimia may evolve into medical complications that will be overlooked unless the clinician is vigilant.

To summarize, with respect to children, looking for psychological masquerade begins with the assumption that significant behavior or psychological symptoms in a child not under significant stress is likely an organic problem. With the exception of reactive depression, a striking decline in school performance is virtually always an indicator of organicity. Psychotic symptoms—any time they appear in children—demand a complete medical workup. The clinician should be sensitive to the association of abnormal movements and "psychological" symptoms in children and should be continuously on the lookout for lapses or "spells" indicative of a seizure disorder. Children with visual or hearing problems may develop behavioral problems out of stress and frustration. The integrity of basic sensory modalities should always be confirmed in child psychiatric cases. Finally, bulimia with all its potential complications is a prime candidate for psychological masquerade.

REFERENCES

Berry, C., Shaywitz, S., & Shaywitz, B. (1985). Girls with attention deficit disorder: A silent minority? A report on behavioral and cognitive characteristics. *Pediatrics, 76,* 801–809.

Caine, E. (1988). Tourett's syndrome in Monroe County school children. *Neurology, 38:* 472–475.

Carethers, M. (1988). Diagnosing vitamin B_{12} deficiency, a common geriatric disorder. *Geriatrics, 43:* 89–112.

Clark, A. (1970). Ectopic tachycardias in the elderly. *Gerontological Clinica, 12,* 203–212.

Comfort, A. (1980). *Practice of Geriatric Psychiatry.* New York: Elsevier.

Cummings, J., Benson, F., & LoVerne, S. (1980). Reversible dementia. *JAMA, 243,* 2434–2439.

Edelbrock, C., Costello, A., & Kessler, M. (1984). Empirical corroboration of attention deficit disorder. *Journal American Academy of Child Psychiatry, 23,* 285–290.

Eisdorfer, C. (1980). Paranoia and schizophrenic disorders in later life. In E. Busse & D. Blazer (Eds.), *Handbook of Geriatric Psychiatry.* New York: Van Nostrand Reinhold Co.

Eisendrath, S., & Sweeney, M., (1987). Toxic neuropsychiatric effects of digoxin at therapeutic serum concentration. *American Journal of Psychiatry, 144:* 506–507.

Fox, J., Topel, J., & Huckman, M. (1975). Dementia in the elderly—a search for treatable illnesses. *Journal of Gerontology, 30,* 557–564.

Friedman, A., Seine, R., Roberts, T., Fremouw, W. (1987). Ipecac abuse: a serious complication in bulimia. *General Hospital Psychiatry, 9,* 225–228.

Golder, G. (1977). Tourette syndrome. *American Journal of Diseases of Children, 131,* 531–534.

Hurtwitz, N. (1969). Predisposing factors in adverse reactions to drugs. *British Medical Journal, 1:* 536–539.

Kurlan, R., & Como, P. (1988). Drug-induced Alzheimerism. *Archives of Neurology, 45:* 356–357.

Laufer, M., & Taranath, S. (1979). Acute and chronic brain syndromes. In J. Noshpitz (Ed.), *Basic Handbook of Child Psychiatry, Vol. 2,* (381–402).

Livingston, S., Pauli, L., & Bruce, I. (1980). Neurological evaluation of the child. In H. Kaplan, A. Freedman, & B. Sadock (eds.), *Comprehensive Textbook of Psychiatry, III,* (pp. 2461–2473).

Lying-Tunnell, V. (1979). Psychotic symptoms in normal pressure hydrocephalus. *Acta Psychiatrica Scandinavia, 59:* 415–419.

Malamud, N. (1975). Organic brain disease mistaken for psychiatric disorder: a clinicopathologic study. In D. Benson & D. Blumer (Eds.), *Psychiatric Aspects of Neurological Disease,* (287–307).

Mark, S., & Gath, A. (1978). *Psychological disorders of children.* Baltimore: Williams and Wilkins Co.

Meller, W., & Lyle, K. (1987). Attention deficit disorder in childhood. *Primary Care, 14,* 745–759.

Mickley, D. (1988). Evaluating common eating disorders—ten questions to ask your patient. *Female Patient, 13,* 33–36.

Ornitz, E., & Ritvo, E. (1976). The syndrome of autism: a critical review. *American Journal of Psychiatry, 133,* 609–621.

Price, T., & Tucker, G. (1977). Psychiatric and behavioral manifestations of normal pressure hydrocephalus. *Journal of Nervous and Mental Disease, 164,* 51–55.

Pygott, F., & Street, D. (1950). Unsuspected treatable organic dementia. *Lancet, i,* 1371.

Raskind, R., & Glover, B. (1972). Chronic subdural hematoma in the elderly: a challenge in diagnosis and treatment. *Journal of the American Geriatric Society, 20,* 330–334.

Reynolds, C., Hoch, C., Kupter, D., Buysse, D., Houck, P., Stack, J., & Campbell, D. (1988). Bedside differentiation of depressive pseudodementia from dementia. *American Journal of Psychiatry, 145:* 1099–1103.

Sacks, O., (1987). *The man who mistook his wife for a hat,* New York: Harper and Row.

Stuteville, P., & Welch, K. (1958). Subdural hematoma in the elderly. *JAMA, 168,* 1445–1449.

Volkmar, F., & Cohen, D. (1988). Neurobiologic aspects of autism. *New England Journal of Medicine, 318,* 1390–1392.

Wender, P. (1987). *The Hyperactive Child, Adolescent, and Adult.* New York: Oxford University Press.

Wells, C. (1979). Pseudodementia. *American Journal of Psychiatry, 136:* 895–900.

Chapter 11

Putting It to the Test:
A Summary and
12 Test Cases

Look to the essence of a thing, whether it be a point of doctrine, of practice, or of interpretation.   —Marcus Aurelius

Psychological symptoms are not always best explained psychologically. Certain organic disorders produce symptoms similar to those associated with psychological reactions. Anxiety, mania, depression, paranoia—these and other "psychological" symptoms can be either psychological responses to problems in living or reflections of mechanical breakdown in the brain itself.

The existence of masquerading organic mental disorders creates a clinical assessment problem for therapists and counselors. As we have seen, studies show that in psychiatric clinic settings roughly one out of every ten patients, if thoroughly examined, has a causative organic disorder. This is to say nothing of organic disorders that, although not causative, significantly aggravate existing psychological reactions.

The clinician above all must retain a "porous" mental set, always allowing for the possibility of psychological masquerade. An active clinical suspicion is the essential starting point for a sound approach to detecting organic mental disorders. To this suspicion must be added clinical familiarity with brain syndrome, a variable constellation of symptoms highly correlated with global brain dysfunction. The four core deficits, one or more of which appear as symptoms of brain syndrome, are:

Disorientation

Recent memory impairment

Diminished reasoning

Sensory indiscrimination

Although brain syndrome usually involves more than one of these core deficits, clinical detection of any of them constitutes presumptive evidence for an organic mental disorder and commits the clinician to seeking additional medical evaluation.

The clinician, however, cannot be content with watching only for brain syndrome; there are other important clues to psychological masquerade. When found in association with psychiatric symptoms, these clues argue strongly for organicity.

We have considered two levels of evidence. Alerting clues sensitize the clinician to the possibility of an organic mental disorder. Presumptive clues are even stronger in their clinical implications; if present, they (like symptoms of brain syndrome) must be considered indicative of organicity. In the presence of psychiatric symptoms, alerting clues include:

No history of similar symptoms

No readily identifiable cause

Age 55 or older

Coexistence of chronic disease

Use of drugs

Presumptive clues are:

Head injury

Change in headache pattern

Visual disturbances

Speech deficits

Abnormal body movements

Sustained deviations in vital signs

Changes in consciousness

Optionally, the clinician can employ three simple screening tests: Write-a-Sentence, Draw-a-Clock, and Copy-a-Three-Dimensional Figure. These tests can be quickly administered. They provide supplemental information about brain functioning.

The search for clues to organic mental disorders need not be intrusive or excessively time-consuming. Through the course of a normal interview, many questions relevant to the question of psychological masquerade will be answered without special questioning. Questions that are not spontaneously answered can be inserted at appropriate points to complete the assessment.

Care should be taken to avoid clinical errors that account for a disproportionately large number of oversights of psychological masquerade.

Mistaking symptoms for their causes

Getting seduced by the story

Equating psychosis with schizophrenia (or functional psychosis)

Relying (unnecessarily) on limited information

Brain tumors (particularly of the frontal and temporal lobes), seizures, endocrine disorders, and AIDS illustrate the range and subtlety of clinical manifestations of organic mental disorders.

Drug-induced masquerades are common. With respect to psychological masquerade, drugs (including medications) should always be suspect. When given in sufficient amounts or in combination with various other drugs, few medications are not capable of causing organic mental disorder. Even the medications used to treat psychiatric conditions have become major perpetrators of "psychological" symptoms in the form of side effects. Both drug intoxication and drug withdrawal can lead to bizarre symptoms easily misconstrued as schizophrenia.

The translation of psychological conflicts into somatic symptoms is called "somatization." This explanatory concept, while often helpful, should be used with caution. Over time many cases initially thought to be instances of somatization prove to be reflections of an organic condition. Certain clinical features of conversion disorder, simple somatization, and Briquet's syndrome (hysteria) are so predictable that when they are absent, the clinician should seriously question the somatization hypothesis.

Old age does not imply senility and should *never* be used as an explanation for psychiatric symptoms. Although diseases such as Alzheimer's and multi-infarct dementia are not reversible, their accurate recognition helps prepare the person as well as his or her family for future complications. It also avoids inappropriate referrals and misdirected therapy. Of even greater importance, a number of conditions easily mistaken for irreversible dementia, if recognized and properly treated in the early stages, prove correctable. This is why psychiatric symptoms first appearing in a person's later years should be thoroughly evaluated medically. Medications should be high on the list of suspects in older people. Sensory deficits, especially impaired hearing and decreased visual acuity, can lead to psychiatric symptoms, as can accidental falls (for which older people are at special risk) by causing subdural hematomas.

As for children, any rapid change in personality or mood (especially if the child appears ill) should be interpreted as organic until a medical evaluation proves otherwise. Other indicators of possible organicity include psychotic symptoms or a substantial decline in school performance.

Seizures and disorders of movement—with their associated psychiatric symptoms—can be mistaken for psychological reactions in children.

Finally, with the dramatic increase in bulimia among adolescent girls, the clinician should be on the lookout for various medical complications.

PUTTING IT TO THE TEST

I have selected twelve clinical cases as a final exercise for the reader. Although most of these are examples of psychological masquerade, some are not; it is left for you to decide.

Your task is to review the cases, taking care to note evidence that argues for the possibility of an organic mental disorder. When you have concluded reading each case, stop and consider the following questions:

What factors, if any, raise the suspicion of an organic mental disorder?

Is the evidence strong enough to merit further medical evaluation?

Based on the evidence, do you think this case was a psychological reaction or an organic mental disorder?

Once you have answered these questions to your satisfaction, turn the page and compare your answers with the known facts.

CASE HISTORY #1: THE TRANSFER

An aging woman in her early seventies was transferred from a nursing home to a hospital for treatment of a urinary tract infection.

Initially, she was managed on a medical service, but within a short time, psychiatric consultation was sought because she was "disturbing the rest of the ward." The examining psychiatrist found her disoriented to time and place. In addition, her general awareness fluctuated widely from one interview to another. At times she referred to objects and people in the hospital as though she were at home.

The patient had been taking several medications before coming to the hospital, one of which was the antipsychotic agent, chlorpromazine. When the psychiatric consultant was unwilling to increase this medication to control the woman's psychosis, the medical staff insisted she be transferred to the psychiatric unit. (DeVaul, 1976)

DISCUSSION: CASE HISTORY #1

Here we have an *elderly* woman taking *medications*, who upon being examined is found to have at least one core manifestation of brain syndrome, *disorientation*. She also evidenced a *fluctuating level of consciousness*. The psychiatric consultant resisted the medical staff's insistence that the woman was schizophrenic and simply required more medication.

After the patient was transferred to the psychiatric unit, all her medications were discontinued. Ten days later she was alert and fully oriented, saying that "she felt better than she had in years."

An interesting additional note: the woman left the hospital to live with her sister instead of returning to the nursing home where she had previously been living.

Medications are always suspect!

Condition: Drug-induced organic mental disorder.

CASE HISTORY #2: WORKAHOLIC

A highly successful businessman, age 45, with no previous history of psychiatric disorder, began to act differently from his usual self. He seemed driven at work. His working hours gradually increased, until finally he was sleeping only 2 to 3 hours a night; the rest of the time, he worked. He became irritable and began to engage in uncharacteristic sprees of spending beyond his means.

Although he felt extremely productive and claimed he was doing the work of five men, the man's boss felt otherwise. He was worried about the quality of his work, having observed several recent examples of poor business decisions.

Finally, when the man complained of headaches, his boss insisted that he seek help. (Jamieson & Wells, 1979)

DISCUSSION: CASE HISTORY #2

This patient had *no previous history* of similar psychiatric symptoms, and his poor business decisions could have indicated a *deterioration in simple problem-solving skills*. But the most compelling evidence for organicity is found in the emergence of *headaches* associated with a change in behavior.

When examined medically, the man was found to have severe papilledema (a sign of increased intracranial pressure detected by ophthalmoscopic examination). Further investigation revealed four tumorous masses in his brain, presumably spread there from another site. Eleven months later, he died of cancer.

Condition: Organic mental disorder secondary to metastatic cancer.

CASE HISTORY #3: THE DESPONDENT LADY

Shortly after the announcement of her only child's engagement, a 53-year-old married woman became irritable and started compulsively overeating. Previously she had been in good health, without history of trauma, alcoholism, or drug abuse.

As the wedding approached, the woman appeared more and more withdrawn. She refused to have anything to do with the wedding preparations.

In subsequent months, she deteriorated mentally. Eventually, she lost her job due to her inability to concentrate. On occasion, her friends observed her obsessively counting out loud to herself. Later, she became extremely fearful of dying and had difficulty sleeping.

She grew depressed and had thoughts of suicide, for which she was hospitalized in a psychiatric facility. Treatment with various psychiatric medications over a period of six months produced no change; in fact, her condition worsened. She then had an episode of catatonia with mutism, after which she was disoriented. Her walking became unsteady, and she began to urinate on herself. (Rosen & Swigar, 1976)

DISCUSSION: CASE HISTORY #3

The stressful life situation is there: A mother, "losing" her only child to marriage, becomes depressed and consequently is fired from her job. Other findings, however, suggest that this explanation might be erroneous.

First, this is a 53-year-old woman with *no previous history of psychiatric problems*. In addition to her becoming depressed, she *loses her ability to concentrate* to the point she can no longer perform her job.

Time and treatment, which usually favorably alter the course of reactive depression, failed to benefit this woman.

The evidence for an organic mental disorder becomes overwhelming when she eventually experiences *catatonia, mutism, disorientation, and urinary incontinence*. Despite these symptoms, this woman was treated with electroconvulsive therapy, during which she manifested additional neurological signs. A special neurological study (pneumoencephalogram) finally provided the diagnosis of normal pressure hydrocephalus. Neurosurgical shunting produced a gradual improvement, but residual symptoms—unsteadiness in walking, decreased spontaneous speech, and intermittent disorientation—persisted, presumably due to irreversible brain damage sustained prior to treatment.

A final note: this woman early in the course of her disease experienced a strong sense of impending death. Although certainly not a universal finding in organic diseases, the fear of imminent destruction often surfaces in association with serious organic mental disorders.

Condition: Organic mental disorder secondary to normal pressure hydrocephalus.

CASE HISTORY #4: "OUT OF THIS WORLD"

"What a curious feeling!" said Alice. "I must be shutting up like a tele-scope!"

And so it was indeed: she was now only ten inches high, and her face brightened up at the thought that she was now the right size for going through the little door into that lovely garden. First, however, she waited for a few minutes to see if she was going to shrink any further: she felt a little nervous about this; "for it might end, you know," said Alice to herself, "in my going out altogether, like a candle. I wonder what I should be like then?"

A while later . . .

"Curiouser and curiouser" cried Alice. (She was so much surprised, that for the moment she quite forgot how to speak good English). "Now I'm opening out like the largest telescope that ever was! Goodbye, feet!" (For when she looked down at her feet, they seemed to be almost out of sight, they were getting so far off.) "Oh, my poor little feet, I wonder who will put on your shoes and stockings for you now, dears? I'm sure I shan't be able! I shall be a great deal too far off to trouble myself about you: you must manage the best way you can"—"but I must be kind to them," thought Alice, "or perhaps they won't walk the way I want to go! Let me see. I'll give them a new pair of boots every Christmas." (Carroll, 1951)

DISCUSSION: CASE HISTORY #4

Of course this is not an actual clinical case history, but rather a quote from Lewis Carroll's *Alice in Wonderland*. I have included it because of Alice's graphic description of her unusual perceptual experiences. She is suddenly gripped by *bizarre distortions in her vision*, alternating between seeing herself first as extremely small and then extremely large.

During this experience, a sense of fear comes over her momentarily and she has *difficulty speaking*.

The history of sudden *changes in consciousness*, if presented by a patient, would constitute presumptive evidence for organicity. More specifically, Alice's problem smacks of the perceptual changes often seen during the initial aura of complex partial seizures. Similar perceptual distortions also occur in rare forms of migraine, a condition suffered by Lewis Carroll himself.

Condition: Organic mental disorder secondary to complex partial seizure (?) migraine (?)

CASE HISTORY #5: DOWNHILL

A 22-year-old male graduate student was referred to the student health service by a professor. Over the past semester, the student's grades had declined dramatically. He found himself unable to concentrate on his studies and had little initiative. He experienced difficulty falling asleep and felt "down" much of the time. These symptoms had emerged shortly after he broke up with his male lover, who had enrolled in college in another state.

Although the young man admitted to the passing thought of suicide, there was little evidence that this was a serious consideration. On examination, he was alert and showed no abnormalities with respect to speech, vision, or movement. He denied the use of medications or drugs other than weekend beer drinking. There was no history of serious injury or disease. His answers to questions revealed an intact, above-average intelligence. (Taylor, 1969)

DISCUSSION: CASE HISTORY #5

This is a case of depression resulting from a significant personal loss; a psychological reaction. The student's poor academic performance reflected a loss of initiative and interest, common accompaniments of feeling depressed. *No presumptive evidence for an organic mental disorder was present.* The absence of such findings in conjunction with an identifiable precipitant argued against an organic mental disorder.

The student was in psychotherapy for eight sessions over a period of two months. By that time he had worked through his personal loss and had resumed most of his social activities. His school performance improved greatly.

Condition: Psychological reactive depression.

CASE HISTORY #6: SUPERNATURAL

Suddenly, she would be "seized by a horrible feeling of terror." These spells came over this 44-year-old woman irrespective of what she was doing at the moment. Initially, she would detect a peculiar odor, "a horrible smell—not a real smell—somewhat like the smell of burning hedges." At times she felt as though she were choking on this unpleasant odor.

Although she rarely lost consciousness, on occasion she fell to the floor. For a short while she would be unable to respond but could follow the conversation going on around her. Sometimes she experienced hallucinations and felt an unusual sensation in her abdomen. (MacRae, 1954)

DISCUSSION: CASE HISTORY #6

Episodic attacks involving a *shift in consciousness, olfactory hallucinations* and the *inability to speak momentarily* must be considered organic until proven otherwise.

When this woman was evaluated neurologically, she was found to be of normal intelligence without memory deficit or disorientation. Visual testing, however, revealed that she was functionally blind in her right eye and had lost the sense of smell in her right nostril. These findings, along with her clinical history, suggested the possibility of a tumor. At surgery a sizable meningioma was removed from the right temporal and frontal areas. Six months later the woman reported that she had not experienced any further attacks. It should be noted that the woman's vague awareness during her seizures easily have been mistaken for a hysterical reaction.

Condition: Organic mental disorder secondary to a meningioma of the right frontal/temporal area.

CASE HISTORY #7: SATAN'S WORK

She was an active high school student, a competitive swimmer, in excellent health. Abruptly, she began to act unlike herself, taking copious notes on her family's conversations and on various television programs. She made comments no one else could understand. At times her speech was jumbled. Three days later, having had chills at night and the feeling that "Satan is taking me over," she was driven to the hospital by her parents and treated with neuroleptic medication, but without improvement. Her speech became slurred; finally, she stopped speaking altogether. Her temperature was 102° F, and she was observed to have a limp. She was transferred to the psychiatric service of a university hospital. (Wilson, 1976)

DISCUSSION: CASE HISTORY #7

A healthy high school student *abruptly becomes psychotic*. She rapidly develops a *speech deficit*, begins to *limp* and has a *fever of 102° F with chills*. The real question is why she was ever admitted to a psychiatric service! Her condition should have been readily recognized as neurological.

Shortly after her admission, a spinal tap showed white cells, indicative of an infection. Her EEG recorded changes consistent with this diagnosis. It was presumed from the clinical picture that she had contracted herpes simplex encephalitis, a viral infection with a particular predilection for the limbic system.

Condition: Organic mental disorder secondary to herpes simplex encephalitis.

CASE HISTORY #8: SUSPICIONS

After six months of alleged sobriety, a 45-year-old woman was admitted to the hospital when she became unable to care for herself. Her husband claimed that she had not returned to her old alcohol habits; nevertheless, she had neglected her housework and had had considerable difficulty moving about the house without falling over the furniture. On occasion, she had lost her way in the neighborhood, and she had been involved in several minor automobile accidents.

While being interviewed at the hospital, the woman claimed that her husband was trying to have her committed so that he could continue his affair with a neighbor's wife. When asked the date, she missed it by 10 days; and later, while on the hospital ward, she wandered away and was unable to find her way back. She made several errors in serially subtracting 7 from 100 and finally declined to continue. Her hands were tremulous. She was only able to recall one out of three objects after a five-minute period. (Horvath, 1979)

DISCUSSION: CASE HISTORY #8

Difficulty walking, combined with *a history of automobile accidents* and *losing her way in the neighborhood* made a psychological explanation for this woman's behavior highly unlikely. The argument for organicity is strengthened by the clinical observations that she was *disoriented* and had a *severe problem with recent memory.*

After several days of hospitalization, a large quantity of proprietary sedatives containing bromides was found in her locker. A blood test for bromide showed a level that fully accounted for her cognitive deficits. Several days later, once the bromide had been excreted from her system, she was bright and alert.

Condition: Organic mental disorder secondary to bromide intoxication.

CASE HISTORY #9: MYSTERY WOMAN

A middle-aged woman was discovered at night in a deserted parking lot by a patrol policeman. She was disheveled and had no possessions with her other than the clothes she wore. She did not speak spontaneously, but did follow simple instructions and made some attempt to answer questions. She had no idea of who or where she was. (Gregory, 1968)

DISCUSSION: CASE HISTORY #9

This woman was found in strange circumstances. She is *mute*. Her untidiness as well as the fact that she appears lost suggest *cognitive impairment*. On this basis, the woman should have received a thorough medical examination.

This was done but revealed no other evidence for organicity. The woman was suffering from a psychological reaction known as a dissociative disorder. Her inability to "remember" where or who she was turned out to be a psychological defense against facing up to having run away. Further evaluation showed that, in fact, she was not disoriented and her memory was intact. Another indicator of the psychological nature of this woman's problem was her disorientation to self. While disorientation to place and time is a hallmark of brain syndrome, disorientation to self is quite rare in organic conditions.

The fact that further evaluation did not confirm this as a case of psychological masquerade does not detract from the importance of suspecting this possibility. Carefully looking for masquerading conditions will inevitably turn up a few false positives.

Condition: Psychological reaction, dissociative disorder.

CASE HISTORY #10: STOPS AND STARTS

For five years a middle-aged man underwent periods of peculiar behavior, lasting from a few minutes to as long as several hours. Gradually these episodes increased in frequency until they were occurring four or five times a week. The man's behavior was quite variable from one episode to another, but always in striking contrast to his usual self.

On one occasion he wandered about his workplace for over two hours, appearing confused; eventually, he inappropriately removed his shirt and stared foolishly at various people who tried to engage him in conversation. During another attack, he abruptly stoped chopping wood and walked through his neighborhood, glassy-eyed, with an ax held in a threatening manner. Finally, when he was taken to a hospital; he spoke indistinctly and exhibited grotesque, purposeless movements.

He had no recollection for these periods which occurred most often after excessive exertion or towards the end of the morning. (Romano & Coon, 1942)

DISCUSSION: CASE HISTORY #10

Unexplained *shifts in consciousness* with a related *memory disturbance*, plus the description, on at least one occasion, of *disturbed speech* and *abnormal body movements* add up to organicity. The fact that these attacks tended to occur after excessive exertion and during the morning hours provides an important clue to the specific problem, hypoglycemia.

Eventually, a fellow employee (whom the patient threatened with a knife during one of these attacks) contributed a detailed description, having observed numerous episodes. He said that the man usually was quite pale, unsteady on his feet, and sweated profusely.

Laboratory studies confirmed that these episodes correlated with severe drops in the patient's blood sugar. The attacks were the product of an insulin-producing tumor, an insulinoma.

Condition: Organic mental disorder secondary to hypoglycemia resulting from an insulinoma.

CASE HISTORY #11:
A THING FOR LIGHT POLES

A 67-year-old woman, a retired x-ray technician, moved to Las Vegas, Nevada to be closer to her son. She was bright, active, in good health, and independent. Her adjustment to her new situation seemed to go well until she started having a peculiar urge. She had never had anything like it before. Now when she would pass light poles on the street, she found herself overcome with the sudden desire to swing herself around the pole and then climb it!

Eventually, there were other changes. When she would leave her house, she felt compelled to crawl through the window rather than going out the door. Although fully aware of the peculiarity of her behavior, she had a hard time resisting these urges. She also started having memory lapses. Events would be completely forgotten. She became disoriented and found herself having to get a newspaper in order to keep up with what week or month it was. Occasionally, she had trouble finding her way home after going shopping. She felt nervous about what was happening. Her intellect, however, didn't seem to suffer. She had no headaches or difficulty walking, and she continued to lead an independent life. (Giarrantano, 1988)

DISCUSSION: CASE HISTORY #11

An older woman undergoes the stress of moving to a new home. She's alone and in a strange place. Is it enough to account for her peculiar symptoms? Not really. Had she become slightly depressed or anxious perhaps so, but not when she abruptly begins to have the irresistible urge to climb light poles and crawl through windows in combination with tell-tale clues of an organic problem.

Although it's true that the ability to remember things normally shows some decline as we age, old age itself does not bring on *memory lapses* where chunks of what has happened are forgotten. She also was periodically *disoriented in time and space*, as evidenced by her having to refer to the paper in order to keep up with the weeks and months and by her periodically wandering off and losing her way.

It's not clear why this woman did not seek help earlier. Perhaps it was her independent nature; perhaps it was her need to deny that anything was wrong. Whatever the case, she suffered in silence for almost a year. Finally, unrelated to her problems, she decided to volunteer as a foster parent. This required that she have a physical examination by a doctor. While undergoing this, she mentioned to the nurse the changes she had been having. The nurse referred her to another doctor. Upon hearing her story, he subsequently sent her to a neurologist. It was only then that a diagnosis was made of a right-sided frontal lobe tumor (most likely a meningioma). The tumor was sizable, but after preliminary cooling, it was successfully surgically removed.

Nine years later, at the age of 76, the woman is a volunteer teacher and a foster grandparent. Her only problem is a slight speech impediment which she developed after surgery.

Condition: Organic mental disorder secondary to a frontal lobe tumor.

CASE HISTORY #12: A RULER'S RUIN

He was a man of considerable power, ruling over a vast empire. Other countries were constant threats to him; but as it turned out, it was not a foreign power that brought down his reign but rather a change in his own person.

In the middle of his life, he began to suffer painful, debilitating episodes that every few years appeared without warning or cause. He would become giddy, talking and pacing about nonstop. His ideas came in torrents; before one was finished, another was taking him on a different tangent. At night his condition worsened. He became confused and began to hear voices and see things that were not actually present. Upon awakening he would insist on seeing the queen to make certain she had not been abducted. On occasion he became exhausted and fell into despair. His muscles weakened so that he could not walk or even speak.

Certain episodes were strikingly different: his body would be racked with pain. He would double over in agony and couldn't stand to be touched, not even by the bedclothes, without raving and crying out.

During one of his most severe attacks, royal physicians debated behind closed doors whether or not he would ever recover his mental faculties. Word leaked out that the ruler was gravely incapacitated. Political forces began to align themselves for a takeover, but suddenly he recovered completely. Several years later, however, he became "violently insane" again. Secret arrangements were made for his wife to assume power. She did, and he remained psychotic with only brief intervals of lucidity until he died nine years later. (Macalpine & Hunter, 1969)

DISCUSSION: CASE HISTORY #12

This is the true story of the tragic life of George III, King of Great Britain during the Seven Years' War when an empire was won, and during the revolutionary war when the American colonies were lost.

In 1941 a leading psychoanalyst, Dr. Manfred Guttmacher, wrote a book entitled *America's Last King: An Interpretation of the Madness of George III* (Guttmacher, 1941). He offered his expert opinion that the King's problems could be fully explained psychologically. "His five manic attacks were precipitated by political and domestic events that pierced his very vulnerable defenses and caused him to decompensate." Guttmacher went on to explain how the King, believing that he should be all-powerful, lost his mental balance "when he found himself impotent and unable to act."

Dr. Guttmacher was wrong. He failed to pay enough attention to certain telltale clues of organic mental disorder. The King suffered *visual and auditory hallucinations*. He became *confused*, more so at night. He manifested a *significant somatic pain syndrome* incompatible with a diagnosis of hysteria or conversion disorder. In addition, he experienced *serious muscle weakness* that prevented him from *walking* and *affected his speech*.

The King's problem was a psychological masquerade. Although to be certain, he had plenty to deal with, his condition was not the result of a stressful life.

Most likely he suffered from an inherited metabolic disease known as *porphyria*. Due to the absence of an enzyme, this condition results from the overproduction of porphyrins, which in turn leads to brain intoxication and organic mental disorder as well as severe attacks of abdominal pain. One-third of persons with this form of porphyria are admitted to mental hospitals, usually with the mistaken diagnosis of schizophrenia or bipolar disorder.

Condition: Organic mental disorder secondary to porphyria.

REFERENCES

Carroll, L. (1951). *Alice in wonderland and other favorites*. New York: Washington Square Press.

DeVaul, R. (1976). Acute organic brain syndrome: clinical considerations. *Texas Medicine, 72,* 51–54.

Giarrantano, S. (1988). Personal communication.

Gregory, I. (1968). *Fundamentals of psychiatry, 2nd Ed.*, p. 352–358. Philadelphia: Saunders.

Guttmacher, M. (1941). *America's last king, an interpretation of the madness of George III.* New York: C. Scribner's & Sons.

Horvath, T. (1979). Organic brain syndromes. In A. Freeman, R. Sack, & P. Berger (Eds.), *Psychiatry for the primary care physician*, p. 228. Baltimore: Williams and Wilkins.

Jamieson, R., & Wells, C. (1979). Manic psychosis in a patient with multiple metastatic brain tumors. *Journal of Clinical Psychiatry, 40*, 280–283.

Macalpine, I. & Hunter, R. (1969). *George III and the mad business.* New York: Pantheon Books.

MacRae, D. (1954). Isolated fear: a temporal lobe aura. *Neurology, 4*, 497–505.

Romano, J., & Coon, G. (1942). Physiologic and psychologic studies in spontaneous hypoglycemia. *Psychosomatic Medicine, 4*, 283–300.

Rosen, H., & Swigar, M. (1976). Depression and normal pressure hydrocephalus. *Journal of Nervous and Mental Disease, 163*, 35–40.

Taylor, R. (1969). Extracted from private clinical files.

Wilson, L. (1976). Viral encephalopathy mimicking functional psychosis. *American Journal of Psychiatry, 133*, 165–170.

Annotated Bibliography

Adams, James L. (1980). *Conceptual Blockbusting: A Guide to Better Ideas*, San Francisco, W. H. Freeman and Company, 2nd Edition.

This is a concise, well-written book on creative problem-solving, with special emphasis on how to create a porous mental set. "Conceptual blocks," says the author, "are mental walls which block the problem-solver from correctly perceiving a problem or conceiving its solution." The greatest barrier to recognizing psychological masquerade is premature closure; being unable to stave off the seduction of favorite clinical hypotheses in order to observe the actual facts of the case.

Ajax, E. J. (1973). The Aphasic Patient (A Practical Review). *Diseases of the Nervous System*, 34:135–142.

The various faces of aphasia are reviewed. The article includes illustrative transcripts of aphasic speech as well as an example of writing produced by a patient with fluent aphasia. There is much useful information contained in this eight-page article.

Anonymous Author (1950). Death of a Mind: A Study in Disintegration. *Lancet, i:* 1–12–1015.

I have quoted extensively from this article in Chapter 3. If I could recommend but one reference to give the clinician a feeling for the progressive emergence of brain syndrome, this would be it. Written by a sympathetic, personally involved, and keen observer, this presentation poignantly communicates the struggle of a deteriorating mind.

Baldessarini, Ross. (1985). *Chemotherapy in Psychiatry*. Cambridge: Harvard University Press. (Revised edition).

A lucid guide to psychotropic drugs. The book includes chapters on antipsychotic agents, lithium, antidepressants and antianxiety medications a well as special topics such as geriatric and pediatric psychopharmacology. The author does a particularly good job of noting potential drug side effects that can be misconstrued as psychological reactions. Given the extensive use of psychotropic drugs, it behooves all clinicians to have a working overview of these substances, their indications, actions, and side effects.

Benson, D. Frank. (1978). Amnesia. *Southern Medical Journal*, 71:1221–1227.

The author characterizes amnesia as the impaired ability to learn despite normal immediate and long-term memory and the preservation of other cognitive abilities. In reading this brief but fully packed article, the clinician will review the various presentations of defective recent memory.

Benson, D. Frank. (1973). Psychiatric Aspects of Aphasia. *British Journal of Psychiatry*, 123:555–566.

Written especially for the clinician, this article focuses on the assessment of impaired language. The author does an excellent job of delineating psychiatric disorders with which aphasia can be easily confused. A number of practical tips are given for distinguishing aphasia from language changes found in psychological reactions. One section focuses specifically on how to distinguish schizophrenic language from aphasia.

Benson, D. Frank and Blumer, Deitrich (Eds.) (1975). *Psychiatric Aspects of Neurological Disease*. New York: Grune & Stratton.

This is a compilation of chapters by different authors, covering the mental concomitants of physical disease, dementia, disorders of verbal expression, personality changes with frontal and temporal lobe disorders, organic brain syndromes, temporal lobe epilepsy, and spontaneous and drug-induced movement disorders seen in psychotic patients. The opening chapter by Normal Geschwind entitled, "Some Common Misconceptions," serves as an excellent introduction to psychological masquerade. The final chapter includes a series of proven cases of "organic brain disease mistaken for psychiatric disorder."

Benson, D. Frank and Geschwind, N. (1975). Psychiatric Conditions Associated with Focal Lesions of the Central Nervous System. *American Handbook of Psychiatry*, 4:208–243.

A comprehensive chapter on localized brain disorders that cause prominent behavioral and psychological changes. A variety of psychiatric symptoms are discussed, including paranoid reactions and visual hallucinations. Specific brain disorders are covered in detail: head injury, brain tumors, syphilis, Huntington's chorea, normal pressure hydrocephalus, and temporal lobe epilepsy. The chapter is extensively referenced (193 inclusions). Although at certain junctures it may provide the therapist or counselor with more detail than he wants, overall, it is an excellent reference.

Comfort, Alex. (1980). *Practice of Geriatric Psychiatry*, New York: Elsevier.

A well-written presentation of the psychiatric problems of the elderly. It includes chapters on the assessment of "senility" and "organic dementing processes." The first chapter is a must; the author does a masterful job in a few pages of introducing the subject of psychiatric symptoms among the aged, placing special emphasis on those resulting from various organic diseases. "Of all old people who present with a 'psychiatric' problem, between 10% and 30% owe their illness to an undiagnosed medical condition, or to the effects of medication, or to both."

Cummings, Jeffrey L. (1988). Organic Psychosis, *Psychosomatics* 29:16–26.

The authors discuss the practical utility of distinguishing between organic and functional disorders: organic disorders require a thorough medical evaluation whereas functional problems require psychological and behavioral interventions. They list specific delusional syndromes reported in organic psychoses including Capgras syndrome, lycanthropy, and parasitosis; and remind us that Schneiderian first-rank symptoms occur in organic mental disorders as well as in schizophrenia and mood disorders.

Duvoisin, Rogers. (1972). Clinical Diagnosis of the Dyskinesias, *Medical Clinics of North America*, 56:1321–1341.

This is a review of various movement aberrations found in neurological diseases. Despite the fact that it is written for clinical neurologists, I would encourage the nonmedical clinician to read this article. Woven through it are quite a number of little gems of clinical observation.

Gelenberg, Alan J. (1976). The Catatonic Syndrome, *Lancet, i*, 1:1339–1341.

A short, but well-documented discussion of the dangers of falling into the clinical trap of always explaining "psychological" symptoms psychologically. The author describes cases of catatonia resulting from Parkinson's disease, viral encephalitis, brain tumors, epilepsy (petit mal), diabetes, psychoactive drug intoxication as well as schizophrenia.

Illowsky, Barbara, Kirch, Darrell. (1988). Polydipsia and Hyponatremia in Psychiatric Patients, *American Journal of Psychiatry*, 145:675–683.

This article provides a comprehensive review of "water intoxication" (from compulsive water drinking) and its various manifestations including confusion, lethargy, and psychosis. It points out that this syndrome has been found in association with schizophrenia, affective disorders, organic brain syndrome, anorexia nervosa, and personality disorders.

Jenike, Michael. (1988). Psychoactive drugs in the elderly: antipsychotics and anxiolytics, *Geriatrics*, 43(9):53–65.

Discusses reasons for the increased susceptibility to side effects of psychoactive drugs experienced by older persons. Includes antipsychotic therapy (and its complications such as extrapyramidal syndromes), anxiolytic therapy, and sleeping medications.

Katon, Wayne, Sheehan, David, & Uhde, Thomas. (1988). Panic disorder: A treatable problem, *Patient Care*, 22(6):148–173.

Presents the different faces of panic disorder including the overwhelming feeling of unreality that the person often feels. Underscores *abrupt onset* as the most distinctive feature. Reviews how patients often sense they are going to die or lose their minds and frantically skip from one health provider to another in search of relief. Phobias, depression, or substance abuse may emerge if effective intervention is not forthcoming.

Lawall, John. (1976). Psychiatric Presentations of Seizure Disorders, *American Journal of Psychiatry*, 133:321–323.

A discussion of the various ways seizure disorders are mistaken for psychological reactions. The author comments on temporal lobe epilepsy as well as grand mal and petit mal seizures and provides three illustrative case histories that "demonstrate some of the principles to keep in mind in diagnosing epilepsy with predominantly psychiatric symptoms."

Lewin, Roger. (1979). *The Nervous System*, Garden City, Anchor Press/Doubleday.

This slim volume is an entertaining and informative presentation of the design of the nervous system. It provides the reader with a relatively painless means of reviewing the neurological underpinnings of organic mental disorders. The author is a superb translator of technical information into readable prose.

Lishman, William. (1978). *Organic Psychiatry: The Psychological Consequences of Cerebral Disorder*, Oxford, Blackwell Scientific Publications.

The most comprehensive single volume on organic mental disorders: an encyclopedic presentation. This is an excellent resource for the clinician wishing to review in detail specific diseases that give rise to organic mental disorders. It is filled with case examples and provides numerous references. The 14 chapters are: Cardinal Psychological Features of Cerebral Disorder; Symptoms and Syndromes with Regional Affiliations; Clinical Assessment; Differential Diagnosis; Head Injury; Cerebral Tumors; Epilepsy; Intracranial Infections; Cerebrovascular Disease; Senile Dementia; Presenile Dementia and Pseudodementia; Endocrine Diseases and Metabolic Disorders; Vitamin Deficiencies; Toxic Disorders; and Other Disorders Affecting the Nervous System. Although not exactly a book for bedtime reading, this is a one-of-a-kind resource of material about organic mental disorder.

Maletzky, Barry. (1973). The Episodic Dyscontrol Syndrome, *Disease of the Nervous System*, 34:178–185.

Relying heavily on his clinical study of 22 persons with episodic dyscontrol, the author discusses this controversial syndrome of periodic violence. Two illustrative case histories are included.

Manschreck, Theo C. (August, 1988). Cocaine Abuse, Medical and Psychopathologic Effects. *Drug Therapy*

Useful overview of the cocaine problem including epidemiology, pharmacology, patterns of abuse, medical toxicity, psychologic effects, concomitant psychopathology, and treatment. Excellent collection of summarizing tables (signs and symptoms of cocaine intoxication, cocaine withdrawal symptoms, characteristics of chronic cocaine abuse, medical complications, etc.)

Meller, William, Lyle, Kim. (1987). Attention Deficit Disorder in Childhood. *Primary Care*, 14:745–759.

Goes over the DSM-III-R criteria for Attention Deficit-Hypersensitivity Disorder. Also covers prevalence, etilogy, diagnosis and management including the possible adverse effects of stimulants.

Moss, Robert, D'Amico, Stephen, Maletta, Gabe. (1987). Mental dysfunction as a sign of organic illness in the elderly, *Geriatrics*, 42 (12): 35–40.

Focuses on three masqueraders found in older adults: Vitamin B deficiency, hypothyroidism, and normal pressure hydrocephalus. Emphasis is on the early onset of psychiatric symptoms in B deficiency, before neurological or hematological changes. Points out that routine thyroid function tests may miss subclinical hypothyroidism in 50% of cases. With respect to normal pressure hydrocephalus, underscores the frequent occurrence of apathy and cognitive difficulty shifting from one task to another.

Perry, Samuel, Jacobsen, Paul. (1986). Neuropsychiatric Manifestations of AIDS-Spectrum Disorders, *Hospital and Community Psychiatry*, 37, 135–142.

Emphasizes that psychological symptoms related to AIDS may be functional or organic. Psychological reactions in response to contracting a fatal and stigmatizing disease are to be expected, but symptoms secondary to opportunistic infections, malignancies of the brain, and direct viral invasion of the nervous system are also common. Presents case histories illustrating these two clusters of psychological symptoms.

Pincus, Jonathan H., & Tucker, Gary J. (1978). *Behavioral Neurology*, (2nd Ed.) New York: Oxford University Press.

Although technical in places, this is a useful reference on selected topics. Chapter 4, "Disorders of Intellectual Functioning," considers several organic conditions seen among children, including autism, minimal brain damage, and nutritional disorders. The concluding chapter, "Distinguishing Neurological and Psychiatric Disorders," contains information on hyperventilation, headache and hysteria.

Restak, Richard. (1979). *The Brain: The Last Frontier*, New York: Warner Brooks.

An extremely well-written and entertaining book on the workings of the brain. For the clinician interested in an informative overview of the neurological substrate of organic mental disorders, this book is essential reading. Although written for a popular audience, it includes fascinating findings from brain research and is amply documented. At well-chosen points, the author confronts the reader with provocative philosophical speculations that further add to the book's overall appeal. It is a treat to read.

Rossman, Phillip L. (1969). Organic Diseases Resembling Functional Disorders, *Hospital Medicine*, 5:72–76.

A discussion based on a study of 130 patients whose initial symptoms led to a variety of psychiatric diagnoses but who subsequently were all found to have organic diseases. The author discusses the futility of trying to match psychiatric symptoms to certain organic diseases. For example, in his study he found that hyperthryoidism masquerades as four different symptoms: anxiety, psychoneurosis, personality disorder, and depressive reaction. This article highlights the need for an *approach to psychological masquerade based on general principles* rather than a cookbook method that assumes that certain psychiatric symptoms will always be associated with specific organic diseases.

Saravay, Stephen, & Koran, Lorrin. (1977). Organic Disease Mistakenly Diagnosed as Psychiatric, *Psychosomatics*, 18, 6–11.

The authors discuss their clinical experience on a psychiatric consultation service, where 4% of all referrals were found to be instances of organic illness masquerading as psychological reactions. Although 4% may seem like a low figure, it is impressive when you consider that these referrals were being made by physicians. The article contains four illustrative case histories.

Stephenson, John, & Ohlrich, Elizabeth. (1988). The Major Complications Associated with Eating Disorders and Their Pathophysiology. Chapter 14 in *Evaluation and Management of Eating Disorders* (Editors, K. Clark, R. Parr, & W. Castelli) Champaign, Illinois: Life Enhancement Publications.

Covers most of the medical problems associated with bulimia and anorexia including cardiovascular and pulmonary complications; gastrointestinal and neurological effects; renal electrolyte, and bone problems. Gives the reader a solid grounding in the medical complications that can be overshadowed by the more dramatic symptoms of an eating disorder.

Thal, Leon. (1988). Dementia Update: Diagnosis and Neuropsychiatric Aspects. *Journal of Clinical Psychiatry*, 49, (Supplement #5) 5–7.

A brief, up-to-date presentation of dementia with emphasis on Alzheimer's disease. Reminds us that early in this disease paranoid delusions may overshadow other cognitive changes.

Waugh, Evelyn. (1957). *The Ordeal of Gilbert Pinfold*, Boston: Little, Brown and Company.

A semi-autobiographical, fictional account of a successful but nerve-racked, middle-aged novelist who sets out on a recuperative trip to Ceylon. As a result of his overindulgence in self-prescribed medications, the gentleman soon finds himself in a terifying world of strange sounds—wild jazz bands, barking dogs, and loud revival meetings—as well as unfamiliar, threatening human voices talking about him. The reader sees the world through the eyes of a man caught up in the throes of the paranoid confusion of organic brain syndrome, unaware of the true nature of his problem. Good reading.

Woodruff, Robert, Goodwin, Donald, & Guze, Samuel. (1979). *Psychiatric Diagnosis*, New York: Oxford University Press (Second edition).

A "no-nonsense," "just-the-facts" treatment of the major psychiatric diagnoses. This book provides excellent discussions of Briquet's syndrome (hysteria) schizophrenia, affective disorders, and brain syndrome. In a time when many psychiatric texts have become voluminous (and often extraneous), this "little" volume remains an excellent practical reference.

Index